Helene Basu, Roland Littlewood,
Arne S. Steinforth (Eds.)

# Spirit & Mind

# Culture, Religion and Psychiatry

edited by

Prof. Dr. Helene Basu
(Münster)

Prof. Dr. Dr. Andreas Heinz
(Charité Berlin)

Prof. Dr. Roland Littlewood
(University College London)

Dr. Arne S. Steinforth
(York University, Toronto)

Volume 1

LIT

# SPIRIT & MIND

Mental Health at the Intersection
of Religion & Psychiatry

edited by

Helene Basu, Roland Littlewood,
Arne S. Steinforth

LIT

Cover image: James Wilce

Printed with support of Fritz-Thyssen-Stiftung

**Bibliographic information published by the Deutsche Nationalbibliothek**
The Deutsche Nationalbibliothek lists this publication in the Deutsche
Nationalbibliografie; detailed bibliographic data are available on the Internet at
http://dnb.d-nb.de.

ISBN 978-3-643-90707-3

© LIT VERLAG Dr. W. Hopf  Berlin  2017
Verlagskontakt:
Fresnostr. 2   D-48159 Münster
Tel. +49 (0) 2 51-62 03 20
E-Mail: lit@lit-verlag.de   http://www.lit-verlag.de

**Auslieferung:**
Deutschland: LIT Verlag Fresnostr. 2, D-48159 Münster
Tel. +49 (0) 2 51-620 32 22, E-Mail: vertrieb@lit-verlag.de
E-Books sind erhältlich unter www.litwebshop.de

# Contents

| | |
|---|---|
| Acknowledgements | vii |
| Contributors | ix |
| Foreword: Madness and Religion<br>*Roland Littlewood* | xv |
| Introduction<br>*Helene Basu and Arne S. Steinforth* | 1 |
| 1  The "Seligman Error" and the Origins of Schizophrenia<br>*Roland Littlewood* | 37 |
| 2  Return of the Religious: Good Shamanism and Bad Exorcism<br>*Andreas Heinz and Anne Pankow* | 57 |
| 3  On the Notion of Social Pathology<br>*Alain Ehrenberg* | 67 |
| 4  The Religious Texture of Experience in Psychosis in India<br>*Ellen Corin and Ramachandran Padmavati* | 89 |
| 5  Collaboration and Collision: The Involvement of Faith-Based Organizations in Mental Health and Suicide Prevention Programs<br>*Gerard Leavey* | 111 |

*Contents*

6 Psychiatry and the Sweat Lodge: Therapeutic Resources for Native American Adolescents 127
*Thomas J. Csordas*

7 Leading and Misleading Religious Boundaries: Lessons from (Mental) Health Seeking Practices in India 141
*Johannes Quack*

8 "Doctor Sickness" or "Pastor Sickness"? Contested Domains of Healing Power in the Treatment of Mental Illness in Kintampo, Ghana 167
*Ursula M. Read*

9 The Person in Between: Discourses on Madness, Money and Magic in Malawi 189
*Arne S. Steinforth*

10 The Experience of Healing and the Healing of Experience in the Pentecostal Movement 207
*Simon Dein*

11 Tradition, Emotion, Healing and the Sacred: Revivalist Lamenting in Finland in Relation to Three Authenticities 227
*James M. Wilce*

12 Healing Enchantment: How Does Angel-Healing Work? 253
*Terhi Utriainen*

Index 275

# Acknowledgements

This volume presents the outcomes of the International Conference on Religion, Healing and Psychiatry held in Münster, Germany, from February 23–25, 2012, which was generously supported by the Fritz Thyssen Foundation, who therefore are especially deserving of our gratitude. In addition, this volume has greatly benefited from the backing provided by the Cluster of Excellence "Religion and Politics in Pre-Modern and Modern Cultures" at the Westfälische Wilhelms-Universität Münster. For that, we would also like to express our appreciation.

A great number of colleagues have further helped this publication along through their innumerable and invaluable contributions during various stages of the conference organization. Among them, our co-organizers Nina Grube, José-Marie Koussemou and Melanie Duch deserve special mention and our most heartfelt and personal thanks. This volume could never have been completed without their commitment.

Moreover, we would like to thank the many conference participants whose insightful contributions set the standard for the high quality of our conference discussions. In addition to all the contributors to this volume, our gratitude goes to those conference presenters whose highly noteworthy papers, for one reason or another, are not represented in this anthology: Hans-Jörg Assion, Ajay Chauhan, Jozef Corveleyn, Peter Ebigbo, Kathy Gandevia, Sushrut Jadhav, Laurence Kirmayer, Wielant Machleidt, Tiago Marques, Harish Naraindas, William Sax and Ekkehard Schröder.

Many colleagues at the Institute of Ethnology at the Westfälische Wilhelms-Universität Münster further supported the conference in the capacity of panel chairs, making Navina Bolla-Bong, Tina Chakravarty, Malte Frye, Pablo Holwitt, Helmar Kurz, Mrinal Patel, Laila Prager, Annika Strauss and Anja Wagner essential assets to the conference proceedings. We very much appreciated your involvement and your input.

But the conference's overall success must also be attributed to the tireless efforts of a great number of undergraduate and graduate students from the Institute of Ethnology and other departments who volunteered their time and passion. Among these helpers too numerous to mention who played a

*Acknowledgements*

crucial role in making this conference work, we would like to point out Melanie Duch, Jens Hagenschneider and Teresa Schüler. To them and all the others: thank you very much!

In the later stages of transforming a number of remarkable essays into a coherent and, we think, equally remarkable publication, we would further like to extend our gratitude to Johannes Zwilling, Rebecca Walsh and Rachel Grace for their tireless and priceless work in editing the manuscript.

And lastly, we would like to thank Michael J. Rainer and everyone at LIT Verlag for their professionalism, patience and flexibility in the realization of this volume.

# Contributors

**Helene Basu** is professor of social anthropology at Westfälische Wilhelms-Universität Münster and is currently acting as head of the department. She is also principal investigator of the project "Mental Health in India" in the Cluster of Excellence "Religion and Politics in Pre-Modern and Modern Cultures" at Westfälische Wilhelms-Universität Münster. The project explores the interface of religion, psychiatry and ritual healing in India. Her earlier projects in India, Pakistan and Tanzania focused on Hindu and Muslim socioreligious practices, possession and identity formations, migration across the Indian Ocean and the "African diaspora" (Sidi) in Gujarat. She has published and edited several books: *Habshi-Sklaven, Sidi-Fakire* (1995); *Von Barden und Königen. Ethnologische Studien zur Göttin und zum Gedächtnis* (2004); *Journeys and Dwellings: Indian Ocean Themes in South Asia* (2008); *Embodying Charisma* (1998). She is coeditor of the *Encyclopedia of Hinduism* (Brill).

**Ellen Corin** is emeritus researcher at the Douglas University Institute for Mental Health and is a retired professor of the Department of Psychiatry and the Department of Anthropology at McGill University, Montreal. She is also as a clinician psychoanalyst and a member of the Montreal Psychoanalytic Society. Her research in Congo, India and Quebec has developed at the crossroad between anthropology and psychology. In the République Démocratique du Congo, she has worked on the cultural coordinates of the person and on therapeutic spirit possession rituals. Her research in Quebec and in South India deals with the subjective experience of psychosis across cultures, and in North India she has worked on limit experiences among ascetics.

**Thomas J. Csordas** is the Dr. James Y. Chan Presidential Chair in Global Health, professor and chair in the Department of Anthropology, director of the Global Health Program and co-director of the Global Health Institute at the University of California, San Diego. He has served as coeditor of *Ethos: Journal of the Society for Psychological Anthropology* (1996–2001), president of the Society for the Anthropology of Religion (1998–2002) and is a member of the American Society for the Study of Religion. His research interests include anthropological theory, comparative religion and medical and psychological anthropology. He has conducted ethnographic research funded by the National Institute of Mental Health on therapeutic process in ritual healing on the Catholic Charismatic Renewal movement, Navajo Indians and adolescent mental health in multiethnic communities in the American Southwest. Among his publications are *The Sacred Self: A Cultural Phenomenology of Charismatic Healing* (1994); *Embodiment and Experience: The Existential Ground of Culture and Self* (1994); *Language, Charisma, and Creativity: Ritual Life in the Catholic Charismatic Renewal* (1997); *Body/Meaning/Healing* (2002); *Transnational Transcendence: Essays on Religion and Globalization* (2009).

**Simon Dein** is a consultant psychiatrist in Essex, UK, specializing in rehabilitation and liaison psychiatry. He holds a PhD in social anthropology from University College London. He is an honorary clinical professor at Durham University, where he runs an MSc in Spirituality, Theology and Health. He has written widely on religion and health among Hasidic Jews, Evangelical Christians and Sunni Muslims in the UK. He is founding editor of the journal *Mental Health, Religion and Culture*. He is chair of the spirituality section of the World Association of Cultural Psychiatry. He is a member of the Royal College of Psychiatrists' Spirituality and Psychiatry SIG Executive Committee.

**Alain Ehrenberg**, a sociologist, is research director emeritus at the CNRS (Centre National de la Recherche Scientifique). He has developed research programs and research units on mental health issues. His main books are about transformations of individualism and autonomy, mainly through the area of mental health: *Le Culte de la performance* (1991); *L'Individu incertain* (1995); *La Fatigue d'être soi: Dépression et société* (1998), which has been translated into six languages; in English: *The Weariness of the Self: Diagnosing the History of Depression in the Contemporary Age* (2009); *La Société du malaise* (2010), which has been translated into Italian and German.

**Andreas Heinz** is professor of psychiatry and director of the Department of Psychiatry and Psychotherapy, Charité Campus Mitte, Berlin. He studied medicine, philosophy and anthropology at the Ruhr-Universität Bochum, Freie Universität Berlin and at Howard University, Washington, DC. He worked with Markku Linnoila and Daniel Weinberger as a special volunteer at the Clinical Brain Disorders Branch, National Institute of

Mental Health. He is a member of the Leopoldina National Academy of Sciences and of the Akademie der Wissenschaften und der Literatur Mainz. He was awarded the Leibniz Chair by the Leibniz Institute for Neurobiology Magdeburg for excellent research in neuroscience and was nominated as Karl-Jaspers Guest Professor at the University of Oldenburg. He also was awarded the Wilhelm-Feuerlein-Award for his studies on serotonergic dysfunction in the disposition and maintenance of alcoholism. His research focuses on dopaminergic and serotonergic neurotransmission and their respective effects on reward-dependent learning, positive and negative mood states and impulsivity. A second research focus is on social exclusion stress and transcultural psychiatry.

**Gerard Leavey** took up the post of director of the Bamford Centre, Ulster University, Northern Ireland, in September 2012. His research career has predominantly focused on mental health services, particularly in the field of illness and help-seeking behavior. Based in socially diverse north London, he has published widely on service pathways and access by minority and disadvantaged populations. His work ranges from epidemiological studies on ethnic elders and refugee children to qualitative investigations of community level agencies such as schools and faith-based organizations and their role in the recognition and management of mental illness. More recently, he has undertaken research on the pastoral work of clergy relating to suicide. In collaboration with Professor John Brewer of Sterling University he explored the religious beliefs and values of ex-combatants involved in the "troubles" in *Ex-Combatants, Religion, and Peace in Northern Ireland* (2013).

**Roland Littlewood** is a Research Fellow at the University College London. He has worked as professor of anthropology and psychiatry at UCL and consultant psychiatrist in London. He was the president of the Royal Anthropological Institute and has conducted fieldwork in Trinidad, Haiti, Lebanon, Italy and (currently) Albania. He has published seven books, four edited volumes and around 200 academic papers.

**Ramachandran Padmavati** is a psychiatrist and a social scientist working in the area of serious mental illness. She is a senior faculty member of the Schizophrenia Research Foundation. As a social scientist, she has worked on the epidemiology of functional psychosis in an urban community, untreated schizophrenia, culture and psychoses and metabolic disorders in mental illness. She has been involved in a number of randomized control trials. She has put in several years of qualitative research in the fields of community perceptions of psychosis, stigma and related issues. She has a published a large number publications in national and international journals such as *Psychological Medicine*, the *British Journal of Psychiatry*, *Indian Journal of Psychiatry* and *International Review of Psychiatry*. She is also a reviewer of many national and international psychiatric journals.

**Anne Pankow** is a psychologist and member of the neuroimaging research group Learning and Cognition at the Department of Psychiatry and Psychotherapy, Charité Campus Mitte, Berlin. She received the Erhard Höpfner Studienpreis for her diploma thesis. She was a scholar at the Berlin School of Mind and Brain and received her PhD in 2014. Since 2013, she has been studying medicine in Berlin. Her research focuses on the investigation of underlying mechanisms of the psychopathology of psychosis. In her recent publication *Aberrant Salience Is Related to Dysfunctional Self-Referential Processing in Psychosis* (2016) she investigates schizophrenia patients and a healthy population with subclinical delusional ideations.

**Johannes Quack** is assistant professor of anthropology at the University of Zurich. His (ethnographic) research interests include popular Hinduism, criticism of religion, therapeutic pluralism, knowledge (trans)formations and biographic and ethnographic methods. He is the author of *Disenchanting India: Organized Rationalism and Criticism of Religion in India* (2012). He coedited the volumes *The Problem of Ritual Efficacy* (2010); *Religion und Kritik in der Moderne* (2012); *Asymmetrical Conversations: Contestations, Circumventions and the Blurring of Therapeutic Boundaries* (2014) and coedits the book series *Religion and Its Others: Studies in Religion, Nonreligion, and Secularity* (De Gruyter).

**Ursula M. Read** worked as an occupational therapist in UK mental health services before receiving a PhD in anthropology at University College London, which was based on an ethnography of family experiences of severe mental illness in Ghana. She is currently a postdoctoral fellow at the Centre de Recherche Médecine, Sciences, Santé, Santé Mentale et Société (CERMES3), Paris, working on an anthropological study of the emergence of rights-based approaches to mental illness in Ghana. Her research interests are in the social experience of mental illness and the ways in which global mental health interventions are constructed and translated on the ground.

**Arne S. Steinforth** received his PhD in social anthropology from the Westfälische Wilhelms-Universität Münster and currently teaches social anthropology at York University, Toronto. His research has focused on discourses on mental disorder, medical diversity and social transformation, ritual healing, cosmology, the occult and power in the context of southern and eastern Africa. He is the author of numerous journal articles and book chapters. His first monograph titled *Troubled Minds: On the Cultural Construction of Mental Disorder and Normality in Southern Malawi* was published in 2009. He also coedited the 2013 volume *Spirits in Politics: Uncertainties of Power and Healing in African Societies* (with Barbara Meier).

**Terhi Utriainen**, PhD, is senior lecturer and adjunct professor in the study of religions and gender studies at the University of Helsinki. Her research and teaching areas include death and dying, gender embodiment, rituals, present-day folk religion and alternative religiosity. She is coeditor of the volumes *Post-Secular Society* (2012) and *Finnish Women Making Religion: Between Ancestors and Angels* (2014).

**James M. Wilce** is professor of anthropology at Northern Arizona University. He has conducted ethnographic fieldwork in Bangladesh, Finland and southwestern United States. Wilce is the founding editor of the book series *Blackwell Studies in Discourse and Culture*. He is also the author of *Eloquence in Trouble: The Poetics and Politics of Complaint in Rural Bangladesh* (2003); *Crying Shame: Metaculture, Modernity and the Exaggerated Death of Lament* (2009); *Language and Emotion* (2009) and numerous articles appearing in journals such as *Current Anthropology*, *Culture, Medicine and Psychiatry*, *Ethos*, *Emotion Review*, *Semiotica*, *American Ethnologist*, *Cultural Anthropology* and *Annual Review of Anthropology*. Together with Janina Fenigsen, he developed the concept of "Emotion Pedagogies," which is the subject of a Special Issue in *Ethos* (2016).

# Foreword

## Madness and Religion

*Roland Littlewood*

Ever since the biblical Hebrews, opponents of new moral and religious movements have accused the enthusiasts of being "mad": acting not only contrary to everyday rationality but with the additional implication that they are frankly insane. To denigrate these movements as insane is to deny them validity. It is to mock their followers for surely only the credulous and simple-minded could take seriously the ravings of madmen? George Bush and Saddam Hussein both attacked the other as "mad," and to explain the Second World War as the conspiracy of a mad dictator is a commonplace barroom conceit in Britain. But when scholars interpret established social institutions such as shamanism as the invariable consequences of "epilepsy, hysteria, fear neurosis, veritable idiocy," or characterize shamans as psychotic and their religion as "organised schizophrenia" (Ackerknecht 1943; Devereux 1956), we may begin to wonder about the motivation behind such descriptions.

Even if they do not seem to have been regarded as particularly sick by their contemporaries, millennial leaders are often described by later academics as insane: Jim Jones of the Peoples Temple; Hong Hiuquan, the leader of the Taiping rebellion; Te Ua, who founded the Maori Hauhau; Evara of the Vaihala Madness; Counselheiro, the inspiration behind the Canudos uprising; England's Joanna Southcott. Scholarly interpretation aside, colonial and national authorities frequently placed the leaders of new religious movements in psychiatric asylums, often as a change from more conventional incarceration: Richard Brothers, George Turner and Sir William Courtenay, the 19th century British sectarians; Ann Girling, the prophet of the New Forest Shakers; Ne Loiag, a leader of Jonfrum in the New Hebrides; Rice Kamanga, founder of the Barotse Twelve Society; Alexander Bedward, the Jamaican revivalist; Leonard Howell, the Rastafarian; Father Divine, prophet of the American sect which bears his name; Elijah Masinde of the Kenyan Dina ya Msambwa; Huynh Phy So, the originator of the Vietnamese Phat Giao Hoa Hoa. In Canada, Douhkobors who demonstrated naked were placed in the local asylum, as were Jehovah's Witnesses in Germany in the 1930s and Pentecostalists more recently in the Soviet Union.

A less impassioned approach might still lead us to examine the links between religion and mental illness. We know that religious preoccupations are common for the person with psychosis, and that the cosmological speculations of schizophrenia frequently resemble those propounded by religious traditions. Is this because of an intrinsic association between religious experience and psychosis—or merely that the larger questions (the future of humankind, the existential crisis of the individual, what is going on?) demand similar, and equally grandiose, interpretations? How can we compare such disparate domains as cosmologies and transcendental experiences with the frank everyday experience of serious mental illness? Can we even place them in some sort of common analytical framework or are they rather modes of thought—personalistic interpretation and naturalistic medicine—which are incommensurate (Littlewood 1993)? This volume seeks to probe these issues and others.

The Westphalian city of Münster remains famous for a brief convulsion in the 16th century when extreme Protestants, fueled by Martin Luther's Reformation, took power in a brief theocratic regime. Their leader, Jan of Leyden, ran naked through the town and burned his bible in proclaiming the simple truth of the spirit within us. (As of course did many others such as the early Quakers of England's Commonwealth republic.) The iron cages in which his tortured body and that of his close Anabaptist followers were exhibited after death still grimly adorn the steeple of the Münster church of St. Lambert (Cohn 1957).

In 2012 a group of psychiatrists and anthropologists met in Münster to reconsider the relationship between spiritual experience, religious doctrine and mental illness. This volume is the result of that meeting, in which the original academic papers are revised through our own debates and arguments.[1] We have presented here contributions emanating from the psychiatric perspective and those from the anthropological and historical. This distinction is perhaps rather vague as many of the participating

---

[1] The International Conference on Religion, Healing and Psychiatry held in Münster, Germany, in 2012 was supported by the Fritz Thyssen Foundation to whom we would like to express our gratitude. For a full overview of the conference contributions, see Basu et al. (2012).

psychiatrists and psychotherapists also had doctorates in social anthropology. And certainly both "sides" had clear sympathy with the approaches of the other.

**References**

Ackerknecht, E. H. 1943 Psychopathology, Primitive Medicine and Primitive Culture. Bulletin of the History of Medicine 14:30–68.

Basu, H., N. Grube, and A. S. Steinforth 2012 Social Anthropology and Transcultural Psychiatry: Contextualizing Multi-Disciplinary Contributions to the International Conference on Religion, Healing, and Psychiatry. Curare 35(1+2):17–28.

Cohn, N. 1957 The Pursuit of the Millennium: Revolutionary Millenarians and Mystical Anarchists of the Middle Ages. London: Secker and Warburg.

Devereux, G. 1956 Normal and Abnormal: The Key Problem in Psychiatric Anthropology. *In* Some Uses of Anthropology, Theoretical and Applied. J. Casagrande and T. Gladwin, eds. Pp. 23–48. Washington, DC: Anthropological Society.

Littlewood, R. 1993 Pathology and Identity. Cambridge: Cambridge University Press.

# Introduction

*Helene Basu and Arne S. Steinforth*

In recent decades mental health has emerged as a widely recognized value calling for worldwide implementation. Overcoming previous conceptions of health as the "absence of suffering," the World Health Organization (WHO) now defines mental health as "a state of complete physical, mental and social well-being and not merely the absence of disease or infirmity" (WHO 2014a). The state of mental health of populations around the world, however, seems to be determined by rising figures of mental illnesses such as depression—in combination with often insufficient state provision of professional care, especially in low-income countries (WHO 2014b).

In contrast to the simple and definite assertions of the meaning of mental health proposed by the WHO and others, earlier works tended to emphasize the complexity and "slipperiness" of the concept as a psychological/psychiatric construction. In 1992 John F. Schumaker noted that his fellow psychologists "have come to view mental health as a composite of emotion, cognition, perception and sensation. In any one person, this composite translates into a pattern of experience and behavior by which to assess that person's overall state of psychological health" (1992:11). It is, however, problematic to draw a clear line between mental health and mental illness, as Schumaker pointed out, since both concepts are "tied to the equally elusive concept of 'normality'" (1992:11). Normality presupposes abnormality, a concept which includes a range of experiences and forms of behavior of personal suffering, or maladaptive behavior, which "interferes with individual and social well-being," causes the individual to lose control and may lead to violations of moral standards (Schumaker 1992:11).

As a medical discipline, psychiatry specializes in translating abnormal experiences and behavior into shifting and proliferating categories of mental disorders, which have since been standardized in the *Diagnostic and Statistical Manual of Mental Disorders* (DSM) and the *International Classification of Diseases* (ICD) in the 20th century. Psychiatry has continued to refine its diagnostic instruments and invent specific methods of clinical treatments—from the asylum and electroconvulsive therapy to chemical medication—in a complex history that can be summarized as a process from coercion to care (e.g., Porter 1987; Shorter 2009).

Conceptualizations of mental health and illness, or normality *versus* abnormality, are complicated in a number of ways. They are bedeviled by historical processes of medicalization and the diversification of the psychiatric field into biological, phenomenological, psychoanalytic and cultural approaches—to name just the most common and broad orientations. They are laden by the *longue durée* of psychiatric institutions that were established under colonial rule in Asia, Africa and other colonized parts of the world and by the contemporary global flows of psychiatric knowledge merging with the neurosciences. Conceptualizations of mental health are inflected by the specificity and diversity of cultural constructions of body and mind and by the normative moral standards of behavior embedded in the social, political and economic situations that frame the lives of selves and collectivities. And, lastly, they are strained by the emergent topicality of the relationship between religion and psychiatry.

The contributions to this volume explore the complexities involved in localizing interactions between religion and psychiatry within discourses of mental health. These are played out in diverse sites, such as in clinical and pastoral care in Ireland and Ghana (see Leavey, Read), in the psychiatric institutions and cosmological rituals of healing in Malawi, India and the US (see Steinforth, Csordas) and in the religious and spiritual practices that have positioned themselves as alternatives to psychiatric care (see Dein, Wilce, Utriainen). Taken together, the chapters in this anthology manifest the great heterogeneity of scholarly perspectives, local human experiences and practical dilemmas constitutive of the borderland where the sick and suffering, mental health professionals and religious actors confront each other. To situate the highly diverse accounts from sites in Europe, North America, Africa and India, along with their respective historical, anthropological and clinical angles, the broader context of the conversation must first be outlined to clarify what is meant by "psychiatry" and "religion."

## Genealogies of Trans/Cultural Psychiatry

Psychiatry and anthropology share historical roots in 19th century evolutionism. The anthropological invention of "primitive society" provided the comparative framework for biological psychiatry's endeavor to build basic categories of mental disorder—associated with the name of Emil Kraepelin—as well as the psychoanalytic theory of neurosis advanced by Sigmund Freud (Young 2003). Freud relied on evolutionist accounts of "primitive society" to construct his model of ontogenetic personality development in which a child recapitulates the stages of phylogenesis by progressing from primitive, magical thinking to reason (Freud 1913). Unlike Freud, Kraepelin—credited in Germany as the founder of "transcultural psychiatry" (Pfeiffer 1994)—sought firsthand (though brief) experiences with "primitive people." Dedicating much attention to whether schizophrenia was a universal disease entity affecting all human societies or a "modern" phenomenon peculiarly linked to "civilized" society (Jilek 1995), Kraepelin famously traveled to Java in 1903, where he spent three months in a Dutch colonial lunatic asylum. While he found that the "primitive Javanese" did experience delusions and hallucinations closely resembling schizophrenia in Europe, Kraepelin proposed that the disorder manifested in "primitive" patients was much milder than in "civilized" ones. In his view, the differences between hallucinating patients in Java and in Germany could be attributed to "the lower stage of intellectual development attained [by the Javanese]" (Bentall 2003:122).

Kraepelin (1918) and Freud (1913) represent the bifurcation of psychiatry into a predominantly somatic and a predominantly psychological branch, focusing respectively on the biology of the brain or the work of the psyche in theorizing mental illness. And although proliferated and diversified forms of psychoanalysis unfolded as influential forces in clinical psychiatry (and in cultural theory) in the US, France, Germany and elsewhere well into the second half of the 20th century, its core theory—Freud's Oedipus complex—evoked much less comparative interest than schizophrenia, the concept at the heart of biological psychiatry.[1]

While anthropologists largely rejected psychoanalytic approaches as fundamentally Eurocentric, the question whether schizophrenia occurred in

---

[1] For classical anthropological debates on the universality of the Oedipus complex, see also Malinowski (1927) and Lévi-Strauss (1955).

"primitive cultures" marked the beginning of intensive interdisciplinary exchange between anthropologists and psychiatrists, initiating an important stage in the emergence of cultural psychiatry. Contrary to Kraepelin, the British physician and anthropologist Charles Seligman (1929) concluded from his observations in New Guinea that psychosis had been unknown in these societies prior to the arrival of Europeans. Although this claim has been contested (see Littlewood), the impact of culture on the occurrence, course and prospect of schizophrenia continues to engage mental health debates (Cohen et al. 2008; WHO 1973).[2] Roland Littlewood and Simon Dein now suggest that religion, especially Christianity, appears as a major factor in the creation of schizophrenia, leading them to investigate the "common evolutionary trajectory" (Dein and Littlewood 2011; Littlewood and Dein 2013) of religion and psychosis.

Unlike psychoanalysis, which tended to decenter dichotomous constructions of (ab)normality, biological psychiatry was tied to institutions of confinement, which, materially and ideologically, underscored boundaries between the mad and the normal. This reductionist perspective of the human mental condition as either healthy or unhealthy, sane or insane, has attracted considerable critique over time—most notably by Michel Foucault (1967), who, pointing to the historical groundedness of psychiatry in the Enlightenment's rationalism mechanisms for the segregation of otherness, considers "madness" a product of society that reflects its own specific normative structure and values. From this perspective, social categories of "mad" behavior and/or experience may therefore be understood as (psychologized) extensions of bio-power, as strategies deployed for "achieving the subjugation of bodies and the control of populations" (Foucault 1978:140).

The historical context of colonialism provides a particularly telling scenario for the pitfalls of psychiatry's cross-cultural applicability. The colonial transfer of psychiatric knowledge to Africa, South Asia and around the globe initiated the establishment of lunatic asylums and laid the foundations of predominantly biologically oriented psychiatric institutions (Bhugra and Littlewood 2001; Ernst 1991; Ernst and Mueller 2010; Sadowsky 1999). In the process, the universalist adaptation of European

---

2  For culturally informed subjective experiences of schizophrenia, see also Jenkins and Barrett (2004).

psychiatric models, categories and techniques to non-European contexts has provided a remarkably instrumental and alarmingly long-lived framework to support the professed superiority of the European mind over the, e.g., "African mind" (Carothers 1954, 1970; McCulloch 1995). By translating cultural difference into essentially racist hierarchies of higher *versus* lower levels of mental development, colonial psychiatry has played a crucial role in conflating images of "insane natives" and "savage madmen" (Gilman 1985; Mahone and Vaughan 2007), after all, "If madness, in Porter's [1987] words, is 'a foreign country', what of madness in a colony?" (Vaughan 1991:101).

Ever since Arthur Kleinman's (1977) call for a "new cross-cultural psychiatry," an interdisciplinary field of cultural psychiatry has emerged which attends to cultural constructions of illness and health, acknowledges difference as a challenge to the universalist claims of psychiatry and uncovers the very cultural embeddedness of psychiatry as a science (Kirmayer 2006; Littlewood 1990, 2000). In its present form "cultural psychiatry is concerned with understanding the impact of social and cultural difference on mental illness and treatment" (Kirmayer and Minas 2000:438); cultural psychiatry draws its own historical evolution from cross-cultural studies on suffering and healing, as well as from clinical endeavors which address the mental health requirements of indigenous, immigrant and refugee populations. Cultural psychiatry is studied by anthropology and sociology in its sociohistorical context (Kirmayer and Minas 2000:438). While this new cultural psychiatry draws on the changing notions of culture as evoked by anthropology—from bounded units to more fluid and mobile cultural practices—both lines of research scrutinize assumptions and the logic of modernity, such as old dichotomies of nature–culture and mind–body (Kirmayer 2006; Littlewood 1990; Sax 2004; Naraindas, Quack and Sax 2014).

Contemporary cultural psychiatry and anthropology often pursue holistic approaches, taking into account cultural constructions of the self and conceptions of illness and health, as well as local and global constellations of power. In this line of thinking, Janis Jenkins (2015) coined the term "extraordinary conditions," which draws together various strands affecting mental illness, personal suffering and general well-being. The term thus brings into view the connections between personal experience, the sociocultural environment and politics:

In the first place, [the term] refers to conditions—illnesses, disorders, syndromes—that are culturally defined as mental illness. However, I also mean conditions—warfare and political violence, domestic violence and abuse, scarcity and neglect of human needs—constituted by social situations and forces of adversity. [Jenkins 2015:1]

Jenkins looks at contemporary psychiatric practices through the lens of subjects with immigrant and non-immigrant backgrounds in the US. She describes, on one hand, the gaps of meaning opening up between what are often stigmatizing psychiatric diagnostic categories and, on the other, indigenous understandings of illness, such as the concept of *nervios*, which Mexican immigrants employ to make sense of suffering (Jenkins 2015; see also Skultans 1997). Understanding the conceptual divergences in culturally informed explanatory models of sickness and the apparent disregard for cultural factors affecting mental illness on the part of mainstream psychiatry are of ongoing concern to what has come to be known as "(trans)cultural psychiatry" (Kirmayer 2013; Kleinman 1980, 1987; Littlewood 1990, 2000; Littlewood and Lipsedge 1985). The emergence of cultural psychiatry in the global north was and is therefore closely linked to migration from the global south and the need to adjust clinical practices to patients expressing experiences of extraordinary conditions in distinctly cultural "idioms of distress" (Bhugra et al. 2010; Bhugra and Gupta 2011; Blom et al. 2015; De Jong and Van Ommeren 2005; Jadhav 2010; Kirmayer 2006; Littlewood and Lipsedge 1997; Nichter 1981). By engaging with classical anthropological research on possession, shamanism and cultural constructions of madness, as well as ritual practices of healing (e.g., Kirmayer 2004; Laderman and Roseman 1996; Silverman 1967), cultural psychiatry contributes to the renewed interest in the possible role of religion in mental health care worldwide (Whitley 2012).

**Religion *versus* Psychiatry**

The relationship between religion and psychiatry is explored in a burgeoning body of literature—not only in cultural psychiatry but also in the theologies, humanities, social sciences, medicine, psychology, anthropology, et cetera (e.g., Bhugra 1996; Blanch 2007; Csordas 1992, 1999; Fulford 1996; Huguelet and Koenig 2009; Jones 2004; Kaiser 2007; Nunley 1994; Schumaker 1992).

In the older anthropological literature, different expressions of religion were assigned to various categories that were, at least partially, ascribed with different degrees of "civilizational" value. Such classifications—often differentiating between formal, official, institutional or organized religion and informal, popular or folk religion (Wald and Calhoun-Brown 2014)—coincided with the analytical differentiation between the universalist "world religions" based on sacred scriptures, such as Buddhism, Christianity, Hinduism, Islam or Judaism and the local, or "traditional" (or even "primitive"), cosmologies (Howells 1948). From the perspective of contemporary anthropology, such an analytical distinction of religious forms based on their degree of institutional organization is a telltale example of social processes maintaining asymmetrical relationships between diverse strands of religiosity, thus suggesting a *quasi* evolutionary supremacy of, e.g., global Christian churches to local possession "cults." Although the concept of "religion" is subjected to numerous, sometimes contested definitions (Asad 1993), the term is used here heuristically to refer to traditions of faith associated with "world religions," local cosmologies and contemporary New Age spirituality.[3]

Even after anthropologists turned to long-term fieldwork, thereby abandoning their models of inevitable unilinear development (yet without giving up their comparative agenda), ideas proposed by the "founding fathers" of psychiatry and psychoanalysis continued to exert an influence on anthropological interpretations of what were now called "traditional" societies (as opposed to the "modern West"). These ideas concerned the interpretation of specific, presumably abnormal forms of experience that were all too easily associated with the alleged premodern world. It has been demonstrated in a vast body of literature, however, that phenomena such as spirit possession are common in past and present sociocultural formations (Bourguignon 1976). While madness is often associated with possession by malign spirits or afflictions of sorcery in different societies, local concepts of madness, possession, et cetera, rarely feature as neat categories denoting any abnormal occurrences as sickness; instead, these concepts tend to be constructed ambiguously: "mad saints" in India are empowered by their madness to act beneficially for others (McDaniel 1989), just as possession may be evaluated in a cultural environment as a

---

3   For a more in-depth discussion on the interaction between religion and spirituality, see Heelas (2005).

positive sign of divinity or as a negative sign of madness and suffering (Basu 2010). Similar observations have been made in various African societies (Luedke and West 2006; Steinforth 2009). But even if "madness" can be attributed to social construction and discourse, such an assessment still requires research and careful application of anthropological methodologies before one may boast of a translation of indigenous categories into the classificatory system of psychiatry (De Jong and Van Ommeren 2005; Edgerton 1966; Goddard 2011).

Historical narratives of psychiatry routinely hint at what psychiatry as a rational medical practice has left behind in Europe—especially notions of possession and witchcraft related to madness. For a long time now, anthropological proponents of the "old" school of cross-cultural psychiatry have shown a peculiar, tacit complicity with the modern critique of possession practices as voiced both within religious and psychiatric discourses (e.g., Fortune 1932). Even when no pathologizing labels were applied to whole cultures—as (in)famously propagated by the Culture and Personality school in the 1930s and 1940s (see Benedict 1934)—religious practices such as those associated with cultural notions of shamanism, witchcraft, possession and exorcism still came to be regularly regarded as expressions of a psychopathological condition (Littlewood 1990; Sax and Weinhold 2010).

At the time of Freud and Kraepelin, religion was thought to have been superseded by science and was therefore rendered irrelevant as a framework for understanding the world in general and issues of human health and well-being in particular. Contrary to this expectation, however, religion has recently been reidentified as one of the key globalizing forces of the contemporary world (Csordas 2009b; Lehmann 2004). At the same time, a global mental health movement has emerged, establishing mental health as one of the most urgent "burdens of disease" at present (Prince et al. 2007). Following the wake of the latter, shifting approximations are now slowly emerging between mental health professionals, theologians and clergy—even as the neurosciences are boosting psychiatry's long contested status as a science on a par with other technology-intensive medical provisions (Rose 2007). Although psychiatry seems to have found assurance of its long sought after natural scientificity, theological and other voices have started rethinking the antagonistic relationship between psychiatry and religion (Bartocci and Littlewood 2004).

*Introduction*

A significant point of entry for contemporary analyses of the relationship between clinical and religious practices of healing is the divergent socio-cultural constructions of human beings or persons (and their "normal" or "abnormal" behavior [Devereux 1956]). The concept of the person, as introduced by Marcel Mauss (1938), encompasses his or her relatedness to the larger culturally constructed social and cosmological forces and is treated as a specific "category of thought" (Mauss 1938). Distinguishing personhood from the more introspective, awareness-focused notion of self, Mauss defines the person as a category of classification related to personal agency and social responsibility. This analytical formulation of the subject in any form of psychiatric intervention is particularly relevant to the comparative study of psychiatries around the globe:

> We see others as persons and experience our own person as a self. While the person may be a category used implicitly in diverse cultures and the experience of self-awareness a human universal, the concept of the self is a hypostatization given central importance in western psychological discourse. [Kirmayer 2007:239–240]

The self of psychology and psychiatry is therefore conceived as an essentially secular person (Rose 1996; Taylor 1989).

**Modernity, Science and Knowledge**

In the complicated relationship between religion and psychiatry, the idea of modernity—of the profoundly "modern" character of science vis-à-vis its "premodern" antagonist religion—has formed a continuous subtext that deserves special attention. In modernist thought, scientific medicine in general and psychiatry in particular are represented as decidedly secular exercises, purified of the old, "premodern" spiritual, magical and/or ritual elements (Favret-Saada 1980; Luhrmann 1989; Meyer and Pels 2003; Styers 2004). At least one influential strand in the current debate on religion and psychiatry thus arises from the modern division of medicine and religion as separate "spheres" (Weber) or "systems" expressing contrary values of secularity and transcendence (Luhrmann). Seen from a post-secular angle, however, dialogue becomes possible between positions previously held to be principally antagonistic.

The relationship between religion and psychiatry thus emerges in manifold constellations and trajectories. A major impetus for the turn toward religion by mental health professionals was the realization that the claims of modernization theory which postulate the decline of religion in a secularized world were incorrect (e.g., Casanova 2007). The transnational flow of Evangelical, Islamic and other religious movements undermine the boundaries between "the West and the Rest" (Csordas 2009a, 2009b; Kendall 2009; Lehmann 2004). Furthermore, it is interesting to note that not only do sociologists and political scientists struggle with what appears to many as a "return" of religion into the public sphere (Brugger and Karayanni 2007; Habermas 2005; Heclo and McClay 2003), but also psychiatrists, who are increasingly reconsidering religion within clinical practice (Boehnlein 2006). The professional worldview of psychiatrists is commonly based on the idea that psychiatry evolved in Europe as the scientific and secular successor of premodern religious, superstitious notions of mental illness (e.g., sin, witchcraft, etc.) (Good 1994; Shorter 1997). At this historical moment, mainstream psychiatrists are increasingly challenged by patients insisting on religious truths and religiosity. Hence the editors of the monumental volume *Religion and Psychiatry: Beyond Boundaries* noted the "long and tense history" of this relationship.

That psychiatry in the twentieth century was largely called a "Godless" period was not to the advantage of the psychiatric patient. Religiosity can be considered a normal personality trait and cannot be disregarded by psychiatrists, whatever their own idea on religiosity might be. [Verhagen et al. 2010:xvii]

While psychiatrists in the global south are striving to close a "mental health gap"—constructing institutionalized psychiatric infrastructures to improve general access to mental health care services in Asian, African and Latin American countries—some of their colleagues in the global north are striving to close a "religiosity gap" to adequately address patients' needs in clinical encounters in the US and Europe. To equip mental health professionals with a better understanding of their patients, the volume presents systematic accounts of Christian (Catholic and Protestant), Jewish, Islamic, Hindu and Buddhist beliefs, along with prescribed religious behavior and conceptions of psychopathology (Verhagen et al. 2010; see also Josephson and Peteet 2004).

The scholars inquiring into the "religiosity gap" in psychiatry represent multiple disciplines, such as psychology, psychoanalysis, religion, the cognitive and neurosciences, philosophy and theology (Verhagen et al. 2010:2). Their concerns partly overlap with and diverge from those of cultural psychiatry, which is directly influenced by its conversation with anthropology. Both approaches worked to ensure the inclusion of the key terms "religion" and "culture" in the fifth edition of the *Diagnostic Statistical Manual* (DSM-V), which was published by the American Psychiatric Association in 2013 (APA 2014; Lim 2013; Peteet et al. 2011). Attitudes of religiosity, cultural understandings of mental distress and diverse constructions of cultural identity brought to the clinical encounter by patients are discussed particularly in regard to diagnostic assessments and treatment. The problem of defining "normal" experience and behavior in terms of varying religious norms and cultural categories, however, is not easily reconciled with the standardized psychiatric notions of scientific classifications of pathology. How can one determine, for instance, whether a person's vision is a mystical experience or a hallucination symptomatic of psychosis? Fulford and Sadler describe the problem as a result of differing worldviews:

Psychiatry, as a discipline within scientific medicine, is at best uneasy with the received authority and revealed truths of religion. Conversely, many of those within religious and spiritual traditions are at best uneasy with the causal (hence deterministic) models of human experience and behavior that underpin the sciences basic to psychiatry. [Fulford and Sadler 2011:229]

From the perspective of cultural psychiatry, however, religion is just as much shaped by cultural discourse as scientific psychiatry. Kleinman decentered the dichotomy between (acultural) science and culture long ago when he asserted that Western psychiatry and non-Western medical traditions both engage in the construction of symbolic meaning-making of (mental) illness, which is then embedded in socially grounded practices of diagnosis and healing (Kleinman 1988).

Many of the tensions between secular and religious worldviews are closely related to a familiar anthropological problem, namely, the opposition between "knowledge" and "belief." In a seminal article drawing on Rodney Needham (1972), Byron Good (1994) demonstrated how "belief" is now associated with error and falsehood. Language, as Good argued, played a major role in intensifying the antagonism between the orthodox Christian understanding of the world as divine creation and the understanding of the world as nature in terms of science. Language became a medium fusing representation with distinct qualities, e.g., in the case of "knowledge" as "holding a correct representation of some aspect of the world" (Good 1994:108). The development of medicine, and psychiatry, was based on the technical language of the biosciences, whose claims addressed factual knowledge of the natural world, not erroneous religious beliefs. Medical anthropological representations of cultural discourses of sickness and healing therefore depicted Asian, African and other phenomena in terms of local "belief" rather than "knowledge." Superior authority and ontological validity was attributed to medicine based on scientific evidence; the knowledge of others was devalued—implicitly or explicitly—and rendered as unfounded "beliefs." In a similar vein—but targeting the ideology of modernity based on the separation of science and religion (or nature and culture) more generally—Bruno Latour summarized the problem in his statement, "A Modern is someone who believes that others believe" (2010:2). Belief, then, is not a state of mind but an asymmetrical relationship shaped by "the work of denunciation" (2010:13). Since Good first formulated his critique 20 years ago, medical anthropology has now largely left behind the old dichotomy between "knowledge" and "belief" (Good et al. 2010).

But the divide between scientific, psychiatric healing and religious or informal healing traditions still exists; scholars and practitioners, however, have suggested various ways to bridge this divide. The theologian Ian Barbour suggested four concepts that can be used to relate "scientific disciplines and their way of thinking, and religious assertions about human nature" (Verhagen et al. 2010:6): (1) conflict, (2) interdependence, (3) dialogue and (4) integration. Integration, for example, draws on recent developments in the neurosciences that bring together science and religion by reconstructing "a religious concept like original sin as a biologically based disposition from the past" (Verhagen et al. 2010:8).

The need for dialogue with not only formal religions but also informal healing practices is stressed in *Psychiatrists and Traditional Healers: Unwitting Partners in Global Mental Health* (Incayawar et al. 2009). The editors echo the familiar secularity constellation, asserting that non-professional healers in non-Western settings would take care of "existential concerns" not addressed by clinical psychiatry, while the latter would advance progress in "understanding the biology of the disease process" among illiterate or less educated populations (Wintrob 2009:1). Moreover, Ronald Wintrob urges psychiatrists to collaborate with traditional healers in "indigenous cultures" in order to "decrease resistance to [psychiatric] treatment" (Wintrob 2009:2).

Given the post-secular understanding of modernity, this call resonates strongly. The World Psychiatric Association now promotes "interdependence," i.e., not the transgression or elision of the long-standing division, but the creation of a bridge between secular psychiatry and religion (Cook 2013; Verhagen et al. 2010; Verhagen and Cook 2010). At stake in this enterprise is not the primarily conceptual consideration of the ontological status of scientific vis-à-vis religious interpretations of health and suffering, but, first and foremost, the needs of those suffering.

Studies are increasingly examining the loss of meaning pertaining to institutionalized religion and the turn toward New Age spiritual movements in Europe and North America (Heelas 2005, 2011; Hervieu-Léger 2004) and Complementary and Alternative Medicine (CAM) (Adler 2002; Naraindas 2011). "Spiritual" healing practices reflect the endeavor to bridge the modern division between secular and religious institutions. The popularity of spiritual healing indicates the downside of the increasingly blurred boundaries between illness and health, or sanity and madness, which Nikolas Rose has attributed to the intervention of the "technologies of life" (Rose 2007). The different spirituality and healing movements express dissatisfaction with the normative, rationalized and impersonal practices of mainstream religious (e.g., Catholic and Protestant churches) and biomedical institutions, placing the individual self and his or her sensual and emotional experiences in the foreground.

## The Volume

While many publications formulate programmatic intentions based largely on scriptural understandings of religion, the contributions to the present volume are mostly concerned with the practical dimensions of the relationship between psychiatry and religion, as well as the challenges and limitations arising from it.

Roland Littlewood (Chapter 1) approaches an early anthropological assertion of the absence of severe mental illness in small-scale, technologically "simpler" societies. As Littlewood argues, explanations of this "error" currently found in romantic and popular science publications declare that only the travails of modernity are responsible for converting the authentic shaman into a schizophrenic; traditional societies, by contrast, have supposedly respected intense and idiosyncratic personal experience, which became subject to reinterpretation in the cultural role of a healer. One such instance is of a religious cult founded by a person who, based on psychiatric criteria, would be considered psychotic; however, in the context of the group, the person is a sane and compassionate leader.

Andreas Heinz and Anne Pankow take up this criticism of romanticism (Chapter 2). The authors proceed critically in light of the current call to integrate religion into psychiatry. The authors draw attention to how psychotic patients were equated with colonized people who were categorized as "primitive" in constructions of mental disorder based on concepts of 19th century evolutionism and modern progress. Ideals of evolutionary development supported the legitimation of colonial violence against "primitive others" outside the European fold and excluded "degenerated others" from "modern societies" (which even reached the extreme of killing those suffering from mental disorder in Nazi Germany). The authors recognize the flip side of the devaluation of the other in the romantic idealization of the contemporary New Age movements of spiritual healing such as "shamanism." However, this may have similar effects of exclusion and discrimination, at least if one considers "the revitalization of [Catholic] exorcism and [New Age shamanistic] therapies against homosexuality," which reinvigorate the conventional Christian norms that had, until only very recently, informed psychiatric and psychoanalytic categorization of homosexuality as a psychopathology in need of therapy.[4]

Theologically oriented psychiatry tends to take "the patient" for granted on the basis of normative constructions of personhood in the sense of the "Western" individual, which are the subject of intense debate and qualification in the field of cross-cultural psychiatry (Kirmayer 2007; Little-

---

4  In Germany, therapists aspiring to become psychoanalysts were barred from practice if they were identified as homosexuals well into the 2000s.

wood, this volume). Individualism, moreover, is not even a uniform configuration of the "West," as Alain Ehrenberg argued in a comparative sociological study of mental health in France and the US (Ehrenberg 2011). Ehrenberg demonstrates how distinct configurations of individualism affect religious and secular articulations of suffering (Chapter 3). Tracing the transformations of the discourse of "social pathology" in contemporary US society, Ehrenberg explores how changes in social norms and values are related to modifications of psychoanalytically defined personality disorders. He builds a subtle argument based on similar patterns of "lament" in 17th century Puritan political sermons (referred to as the "American jeremiad") and in contemporary complaints about the weakening of social bonds of cohesion (e.g., family), of experiences of loneliness and of increasing pressure from the workplace for the individual to be self-reliant and perform successfully. Ehrenberg shows how the demands placed on the individual correspond to the shifting psychoanalytic narratives of psychic suffering, hence shaping the modern conception of the self: "transference neurosis" based on psycho-dynamic conflict is giving way to "character neurosis" (narcissistic disorders), i.e., problems of the ideal ego and feelings of inadequacies and loss (depression). According to Ehrenberg, social pathology is to be understood in terms of the society's hierarchy of values: personal autonomy has become the paramount value and social relatedness has become secondary. But since social relationships are increasingly being formulated in a language of affect and emotion, the value of social relatedness can only be articulated through individual psychological suffering. Mental health and suffering are therefore both revealed as secular language games generating and continuously transforming what Durkheim (1933) called the "modern cult of the individual."

Ellen Corin and Ramachandran Padmavati (Chapter 4) use a comparative perspective to explore subjective experiences of persons diagnosed with psychosis in India. They argue that an interpretation of schizophrenia has to take into account not only the personal experiences and resources of the patient but also the wider cultural, and in this case religious, meanings through which the condition is expressed. The significance of religion for Indian patients is compared with its significance for Canadian patients suffering from psychosis. A subtle analysis is presented of the ways in which Indian patients resort to religious signifiers that seem much less relevant to their Canadian counterparts. Indian society is marked by religious plurality and the deep entanglement of everyday life with religious values and practices. The authors elaborate how psychotic patients draw on religious signifiers, often taken from other traditions, to give meaning to their experiences of alienation and inner turmoil. Two Indian patients are described: one is Muslim, but has appropriated Christian religious symbols and figures to make sense of his schizophrenia, and the other integrates Christian and Hindu themes more idiosyncratically; his experience itself is a clear manifestation of these new themes. The authors claim that sufferers turn to religion as a way to regard the loss of everyday sensual reality accompanying schizophrenia. But religious articulations do not necessarily lead to the patient's reintegration into the family. Family members of psychotic patients may take them to religious places, or to exorcisms, but this does not mean that they share an understanding of religious symbols. While religion may be seen as providing a "palette of resources" that can be applied in very different ways, patient narratives "open to a blurred reality where the distinctions between 'sane' and 'pathological' in the use of religious references often get obscured."

Gerard Leavey examines cooperation between mental health professionals and ministers, as well as the practical challenges involved in such relationships (Chapter 5). In particular he discusses the results of an empirical study of suicide prevention in Ireland, in which Christian clergy and mental health professionals were asked to cooperate by the government. In his nuanced analysis, Leavey unravels the strands of friction elicited by confrontation with the most extreme manifestation of mental suffering: suicide.

For centuries, Christianity has marked suicide as one of the gravest possible sins to be committed by humans. The clergy thus face moral and ideological conflicts when asked by the Irish government to provide mental health services in this context. Although the official attitude of the Church has softened somewhat (e.g., they no longer deny suicides a "Christian burial"), there is no "universal theological stance on suicide and mental illness," as Leavey points out, to guide pastoral care in secular mental health care services. Moreover, suspicions that psychiatric practitioners continue to pathologize their religion loom large among religious professionals. The long history of medicalization of emotions cannot be undone voluntarily but lives on in the feelings of the clergy, who feel that their spiritual knowledge is undervalued by psychology and psychiatry and that their spiritual care is strangely irrelevant and far removed from the problems they are asked to address.

Based on his research in a North American setting, Thomas Csordas (Chapter 6) explores cooperation between psychiatry and Navaho practices of healing mental distress. He presents an ethnographic account of the integration of indigenous practices of healing into an inpatient psychiatric unit treating American Indian adolescents in the US. The establishment of the unit testifies to the increasing recognition of indigenous healing practices, which are no longer viewed as manifestations of superstitious beliefs but constitute forms of knowledge in treating "mental illness." Csordas considers psychiatry and indigenous practices as a repertoire of healing, "a reservoir of cultural resources," for persons to cope with "serious emotional, cognitive and behavioral disturbance[s]." In practice, however, the various resources provided by psychiatry (e.g., different forms of therapy, psychoactive medication) may intersect or clash with the resources of indigenous healing modalities. In his nuanced analysis, Csordas draws on techniques of the body and the theory of embodiment, which allow him to delineate intersections (e.g., psychotherapeutic and Native American notions of "growth"), as well as clashes (e.g., local rejection of psychiatric medication in favor of herbal medicines).

Johannes Quack shifts the focus from psychiatrists to health seekers (Chapter 7). Grounded in ethnographic research conducted in a psychiatric unit in a North Indian hospital, Quack challenges the construction of the relationship between psychiatric and ritual healing in terms of "secular" and "religious" therapeutic modalities. He observes that patients undergoing psychiatric treatment often seek help from ritual healers at the same time and inquires into the significance of religious boundaries when people decide on a cure. Reflecting on the problematic and contested nature of the term "religion," Quack suggests focusing on a person's religious actions rather than a reified "system" of religion. Different ways of "interpreting and living" religiosity are revealed from such an approach. These modes account for actions that oscillate between overtly stressing religious boundaries to ignoring them in certain situations, e.g., when the patient's wish to get well is more important than the religious identity of the healer or the healing place.

Ursula Read elaborates on this complex situation in terms of mental health professionals in Ghana, who find themselves in competition for authority and powers of healing with Pentecostal, Muslim and local practitioners (Chapter 8). Observing that the patterns of disordered behavior, thought and social functioning recognized as manifestations of madness in her Ghanaian setting bear some resemblance to the psychiatric categories of schizophrenia and psychosis, she looks closely at the locally employed ways of coping and health seeking. While popular discourses tend to relate madness to notions of spirit possession or witchcraft, Read's rich ethnographic data reveal a much more non-dualistic approach to severe mental illness as displayed by the afflicted persons themselves and those who care for them. Accordingly, the Ghanaian health seekers represented in her study do not follow the logic of classifying their condition in either psychiatric or religious terms—as either psychosis or "possession madness," respectively—but stress the uncertainties and indeterminacies "around the causation of illness and a lack of systematization in approaches to healing." Moreover, many of her counterparts were skeptical of the effectiveness of the healing practices, thereby stressing the evaluative and strongly pragmatic perspective of individual actors. Given the unpredictable nature of psychosis, the main concern of health seekers appears to be finding a cure that enables them to adapt to the challenges posed to both patients and their families by a disorder that "comes and goes."

This juxtaposition of psychiatry alongside essentially religious ideas and practices challenges the previous theoretical approaches that argued for the conceptual distinctiveness of scientific knowledge in opposition to other, implicitly less validated epistemologies. Arne Steinforth explores the relationships between psychiatry and religion through the lens of notions of personhood and their transformation in Malawi (Chapter 9). Focusing on the effects of global transfers of psychiatric knowledge on local ideas of personhood and, accordingly, on the social relevance of cosmological discourses on psychiatry and mental disorder, he begins by analyzing the concept of the individual and its association with European social structures (which are also, as Ehrenberg argues elsewhere in this volume, strongly North American). By virtue of the strong conceptual ties between secularized individualism and the psychiatric analytical tools of psychiatry, Steinforth questions how psychiatric services should address mental disorder in societies where religious conceptions of the self are predominant. He investigates the rise of the neoliberal economy alongside the perceived increase of secret ritual techniques (witchcraft) applied in the *quasi* individualistic pursuit of personal economic success and their links to local discourses of mental disorder. Within the context of ongoing social transformation in Malawi, Steinforth proposes that two levels of analysis must be distinguished: the concept of the individual person, as well as the analytical others, e.g., notions of the "relational" or "dividual" self (Marriott 1976; Robbins 2002; Strathern 1988) and the specific social values. If values are seen as defining persons and their perspectives on mental health and healing, then there is not only more specific means of analyzing social difference but also a more dynamic, integrative approach for conceptualizing plural models of personhood, psychiatry and healing in Africa, Europe and beyond.

Pentecostalism has long been recognized as one of the most visible contemporary religious movements; it circulates in networks of loosely connected churches all around the globe, individualizing selves through healing (Brison 2002; Corten and Marshall-Fratani 2001; Kray 2002; Leavey 2004; Maxwell 1998; Meyer 2002). Setting off from the relative neglect shown by scholars of religion to experiences of the body (Ahlbäck and Dahla 2001), Simon Dein (Chapter 10) inquires into the work of Pentecostal healing and highlights the attention directed at sensual and embodied religious experiences. Focusing on the explanatory models of demonic disorder constructed in Pentecostal discourses of illness, Dein delineates the ambiguous and shifting attitudes maintained by priests regarding biomedical or psychiatric models of mental disorder. Rather than outwardly rejecting the latter, Pentecostalism accommodates biomedical practices, thereby straddling the boundary between religion and medicine in its everyday practice.

Similarly concerned with transcending the division between tradition and modernity, or religion and secularity, Jim Wilce (Chapter 11) explores the translation of the Karelian tradition of lamenting into new therapeutic practices, which target the release of emotional experiences and expressions, in contemporary Finland. The link between "old" and "traditional" or "new" and "modern" forms of performances of lament is emphasized in the idea of the authenticity of healing, which may reflect adherence to interactions between "the human performer and an entity whose capacity is to bless/heal or curse," or the psychological truth of the experience for participants and their spiritual efficacy.

In her chapter on angel healing in Finland, Terhi Utriainen (Chapter 12) addresses the phenomenon of mixing conventional Christian concepts (i.e., angels) with New Age practices (e.g., Reiki). Leaving behind the pastoral care and secular therapies in a "post-secular" world, the participants in her ethnographic research did not turn to angels because they "believed" in them but because they provided a sense of empowerment. Angels are metaphors made in practices of healing; their agency helped participants overcome, rather than succumb to, subjective feelings of depression and experiences of emotional crises. Drawing on Latour's (2007) notion of actor networks, which are constituted by the assemblage of human and non-human agents, Utriainen argues that the practice of angel healing "highlights relational and participatory agency" and cannot be reduced to the individual self of modernist ideology. By focusing on networks of agency, anthropologists can overcome the opposition between "modern" and "traditional" practices of healing. New Age angel healing is hence analogous to possession healing, which is being analyzed by anthropologists elsewhere in the world, such as India (Basu 2014; Sax 2009).

These contributions exemplify a specific analytic approach embedded in a broader field of interdisciplinary inquiry. The focus on deep ethnographic descriptions reveals how global flows of psychiatric knowledge and institutions, historically and culturally localized, are contributing to ongoing processes of diversification of "mental health" across the global north and south. From diverse analytic angles, an overview is provided of some of the issues situated at the interface of religion and psychiatry in historical and contemporary anthropological research.

**Religion and Psychiatry: Mental Health Beyond Binaries?**

The present volume reflects the ongoing competition between psychiatry and religion, which is investigated from an array of situated perspectives, i.e., the perspectives of clinicians and patients, of healers and sufferers. Many contributors are critical of the boundary between "modern" psychiatry and "traditional" forms of healing; they are also critical of the preeminence of psychiatric knowledge and the need for "traditional" or religious healers to become skilled in this area. Religious and psychiatric models may instead afford viable cosmological frameworks for understanding suffering and healing, causality and redemption—conveying an overarching idea of what it is to be human. If religion may indeed be described as therapeutic, this may be due to its capacity to enlist transcendent forces from the cosmological realm beyond the suffering person. To alleviate the distress of both the unhappy and the insane, such forces from another world—referred to as spirits and divinities in the existing religious repertoire—derive their power from being "other": transcendent, spiritual or even scientific. In a disenchanted world, new therapeutic agencies, derived from natural energies or from revitalized figures of religious tradition, serve to guide and assist the suffering person. In many of the settings addressed throughout this volume, locally recognized practitioners do not tap into the scholarly idiom of what could be regarded as "a religion" but employ pragmatic bits and pieces of everyday "spiritual" understanding—partially novel and ancient, partially familiar and foreign—that continue to be relevant in the social lives of their communities. In the end, therapeutic efficacy does not seem to depend on conformity with some accepted and established religious dogma, but on whether it brings about a more satisfactory, meaningful state of being. The mediating figures, the powerful cultural symbols summoned to assist in this endeavor—whether professional psychiatrists, energies of the natural world, spirits of the dead, deities or saints, the recovered sufferers or projections of the psyche—may all provide healing and redemption. Therapeutic possibility alone is the moral imperative.

Among its many dimensions, the conceptual (dis)juncture between essentially religious notions of the spirit vis-à-vis more psychiatrically valid ideas of the mind must also be recognized as a field of contested claims of authority and knowledge. The ideological and, importantly, often hierarchical concepts that corroborate the distinction between different approaches to mental health are, however, subject to change, critique and contestation. In this context, the ostensibly self-evident discordancy between religion and psychiatry—a collision of competing ideologies defining the normal *versus* abnormal human condition—draws attention to larger flows of ideas, the global transfer of psychiatric knowledge and the role of ongoing processes of social transformation.

With the growing realization that recent transnational developments toward modernization have not given rise to a more uniformly secular orientation of all societies (as classical modernization theory had long anticipated), the competitive "game of truth" between scientific and non-scientific approaches in psychiatry can no longer be understood in geographical terms, or, for that matter, as a division between avowedly modern and allegedly traditional social arenas. Rather, lines are drawn, diffused and shifting in the centers of societies (and in persons) themselves, creating complex pluralistic landscapes of healing in which personal values, experience, aspirations and agency become central landmarks.

Colonial and postcolonial transfers of psychiatric knowledge strongly resemble the dissemination of Christian ideas throughout the world, especially regarding claims of universal validity and truth. Both psychiatry and established Christian churches form powerful global networks that materialize in local contexts. The pluralized landscapes of medical and religious traditions in these settings become asymmetrically juxtaposed to biomedicine, leading psychiatry to coexist as one among multiple—yet often the most privileged—discourses of understanding of mental disorder.

Following the work of Foucault, anthropologists and historians working in diverse cultural settings have demonstrated how the global expansion of psychiatric discourse has resulted in the invention of new pathologies and in the medicalization of emotions, non-normative behavior and abnormal experience (Horwitz and Wakefield 2007; Leckie 2004; Whyte 1989; Young 2005). Such scholars inspired by Foucault share with sociologists of modernization the emphasis on processes of medicalization as forms of social control. The former conceive of medicalization in terms of techniques of governing, whereas the latter stress the replacement of "traditional" institutions of religion with mental health (Conrad 1992; Lock 2004; Scull 1991; Wilce 2004). While the anthropology of psychiatry's emphasis on social control tended to foster the polarization of perspectives in the 1980s and 1990s, more recent studies not only demonstrate the great degree of diversity among local traditions of psychiatry but have also found that the impact of psychiatry is far less linear and unidirectional than previously presumed (Béhague 2008; Gaines 1992; Luhrmann 2000; Young 2008). This is particularly apparent in the complex relationship between psychiatry and religion, as well as in the perspectives taken by health-seeking persons.

In this context, a number of chapters in this volume focus on the person as a fundamentally empowered agent who transcends conventional institutional dichotomies, counteracts prevalent assumptions, negotiates cosmological uncertainties and redefines socially constructed realities on the basis of emotional experience, shifting value systems and a high measure of ambiguity tolerance. These conflicting epistemologies of healing and the nature of the negotiations between them draw attention to issues of personhood, the uneven influence of secularized notions of the individual, the emergence (and renunciation) of the neoliberal economy and its values, the inconsistencies of belief and behavior, the efficiency and experience of non-human agency, emotion and the authenticity of healing, postsecular amalgamations of healing concepts and fading dichotomies between "old" and "new" psychiatric practices. Consequently, this argues for a more differentiated view of the pervasive interconnections between religion and psychiatry which are enacted in human actions informed by ideological models of rationalization on the one hand and emotional responses to lived experience on the other.

The line of inquiry followed in this volume addresses how the poles of biologized science and religion are emerging as intertwined with social and cultural practices, not separate realms or autonomous systems of knowledge. Modern institutions, however, are built on processes that separate fields (e.g., medicine is separated from religion), which are conceptualized by Latour as "practices of purification" (Latour 1991). Straddling the overlap between two allegedly distinct social spheres, the interface between religion and psychiatry discussed throughout this volume reflects what James Clifford described as a cultural contact zone: "[A] contact perspective emphasis[ing] how subjects are constituted in and by their relations to each other. [It stresses] co-presence, interaction, interlocking understandings and practices, often with radically asymmetrical relations of power" (Clifford 1997:192). Here, we are concerned with simultaneous processes of unsettling boundaries between well-being and suffering in contemporary psychiatric discourses, on the one hand, and religious discourses of madness and possession as the subject of medicalization and separations (Latour's "purification"), on the other. Both processes mirror practical circumventions of the division separating secular and religious understandings of healing and affliction.

Numerous important and related aspects were outside of the immediate scope of this volume: Since issues concerning the social lives of psychopharmaceuticals (Jenkins 2011) or the role of religion in global mental health policy are not addressed extensively by the contributors here, they should be taken up in future research. Taking account of the shifting meanings of "religion" in global modernities, the contributions to this anthology reveal how historically and culturally embedded local encounters between psychiatry, religious experience and ritual healing contribute to an increasing diversification of "mental health." The diverse theoretical perspectives and methodological approaches presented here concerning the global north and south introduce novel insights into current debates between clinical practitioners, ethnographic fieldworkers and historians of psychiatry.

**References**

Adler, S. R. 2002 Integrative Medicine and Culture: Toward an Anthropology of CAM. Medical Anthropological Quarterly 16(4):412–414.

Ahlbäck, T., and B. Dahla, eds. 2001 Religion and the Body. Abo: Donner Institute for Research in Religious and Cultural History.

APA 2014 DSM-5 Implementation and Support. dsm5.org/Pages/Default.aspx.

Asad, T. 1993 Genealogies of Religion. Baltimore: John Hopkins University Press.

Bartocci, G., and R. Littlewood 2004 Modern Techniques of the Supernatural: A Syncretism between Miraculous Healing and the Mass Media. Social Theory & Health 2:18–28.

Basu, H. 2009 Contested Practices of Control: Psychiatric and Religious Mental Health Care in India. Curare 32(1+2):28–39.

———. 2010 Healing Madness through Ritual Trials. In Histories of Intimacy and Situated Ethnography. K. I. Leonard, G. Reddy, and A. G. Gold, eds. Pp. 215–238. Delhi: Manohar.

———. 2014 Dava and Dua: Negotiating Psychiatry and Ritual Healing of Madness. In Asymmetrical Conversations: Contestations, Circumventions, and the Blurring of Therapeutic Boundaries. H. Naraindas, J. Quack, and W. Sax, eds. Pp. 162–199. Oxford: Berghahn.

Béhague, D. P. 2008 The Domains of Psychiatric Practice: From Centre to Periphery. Culture, Medicine and Psychiatry 32:140–151.

Benedict, R. 1934 Patterns of Culture. Boston: Houghton Mifflin Company.

Bentall, R. P. 2003 Madness Explained: Psychosis and Human Nature. London: Penguin Books.

Berner, U., and J. Quack, eds. 2012 Religion und Kritik in der Moderne. Berlin: LIT Verlag.

Bhugra, D. 1996 Psychiatry and Religion: Context, Consensus and Controversies. London: Routledge.

Bhugra, D., T. Craig, and K. Bhui 2010 Mental Health of Refugees and Asylum Seekers. Oxford: Oxford University Press.

Bhugra, D., and S. Gupta, eds. 2011 Migration and Mental Health. Cambridge: Cambridge University Press.

Bhugra, D., and R. Littlewood, eds. 2001 Colonialism and Psychiatry. Delhi: Oxford University Press.

Bibeau, G., and E. Corin 2010 Dr Ravi L. Kapur (1938–2006): A Psychiatrist at the Crossroads of Multiple Worlds. Transcultural Psychiatry 47(1):159–180.

Blanch, A. 2007 Integrating Religion and Spirituality in Mental Health: The Promise and the Challenge. Psychiatric Rehabilitation Journal 30(4):251–260.

Blom, J. D., I. T. Poulina, T. L. van Gellecum, and H. W. Hoek 2015 Traditional Healing Practices Originating in Aruba, Bonaire, and Curaçao: A Review of the Literature on Psychiatry and Brua. Transcultural Psychiatry 52(6):840–860.

Boehnlein, J. K. 2006 Religion and Spirituality in Psychiatric Care: Looking Back, Looking Ahead. Transcultural Psychiatry 43(4):634–651.

Bourguignon, E. 1976 Possession. San Francisco: Sandler and Sharp.

Brison, K. J. 2002 Crafting Sociocentric Selves in Religious Discourse in Fiji. Ethos 29(4):453–474.

Brugger, W., and M. M. Karayanni 2007 Religion in the Public Sphere: A Comparative Analysis of German, Israeli, American and International Law. New York: Springer.

Carothers, J. C. 1954 The Psychology of Mau Mau: Colony and Protectorate of Kenya. Nairobi: Government Press.

———. 1970 The African Mind in Health and Disease: A Study in Ethnopsychiatry. New York: Negro Universities Press.

Carstairs, G. M., and R. L. Kapur 1976 The Great Universe of Kota: Stress, Change and Mental Disorder in an Indian Village. London: Hogarth Press.

Casanova, J. 2007 Rethinking Secularization: A Global Comparative Perspective. *In* Religion, Globalization, and Culture. P. Beyer and L. Beaman, eds. Pp. 101–120. Leiden: Brill.

Clifford, J. 1997 Routes: Travel and Translation in the Late Twentieth Century. Cambridge, MA: Harvard University Press.

Cohen, A., V. Patel, and O. Gureje 2008 Questioning an Axiom: Better Prognosis for Schizophrenia in the Developing World? Schizophrenia Bulletin 34(2):299–344.

Conrad, P. 1992 Medicalization and Social Control. Annual Review of Sociology 18:209–232.

Cook, C. C. H. 2013 Recommendations for Psychiatrists on Spirituality and Religion. London: Royal College of Psychiatrists.

Corten, A., and R. Marshall-Fratani 2001 Between Babel and Pentecost: Transnational Pentecostalism in Africa and Latin America. London: Hurst.

Csordas, T. J. 1992 The Affliction of Martin: Religious, Clinical and Phenomenological Meaning in a Case of Demonic Oppression. *In* Ethnopsychiatry: The Cultural Construction of Professional and Folk Psychiatry. A. D. Gaines, ed. Pp. 125–169. Albany: State University of New York Press.

———. 1999 Body/Meaning/Healing. New York: Palgrave Macmillan.

———. 2009a Global Religion and the Reenchantment of the World: The Case of the Catholic Charismatic Renewal. *In* Transnational Transcendence: Essays on Religion and Globalization. T.J. Csordas, ed. Pp. 73–96. Berkeley: University of California Press.

———. ed. 2009b Transnational Transcendence: Essays on Religion and Globalization. Berkeley: University of California Press.

Davar, B. 2015 Justice in Erwadi: A Case Study. *In* The Law of Possession: Ritual, Healing, and the Secular State. H. Basu and W. S. Sax, eds. Pp. 117–137. Oxford: Oxford University Press.

De Jong, J. T. V. M., and M. van Ommeren 2005 Mental Health Services in a Multicultural Society: Interculturalization and its Quality Surveillance. Transcultural Psychiatry 42(3):437–456.

Dein, S. 2008 Jinn, Psychiatry and Contested Notions of Misfortune among East London Bangladeshis. Transcultural Psychiatry 45(1):31–55.

Dein, S., and R. Littlewood 2007 The Voice of God. Anthropology & Medicine 14(2):213–228.

———. 2011 Religion and Psychosis: A Common Evolutionary Trajectory? Transcultural Psychiatry 48(3):318–335.

Devereux, G. 1956 Normal and Abnormal: The Key Problem in Psychiatric Anthropology. *In* Some Uses of Anthropology, Theoretical and Applied. J. Casagrande and T. Gladwin, eds. Washington: Anthropological Society.

Durkheim, É. 1933 The Division of Labor in Society. New York: Free Press.

Edgerton, R. 1966 Conceptions of Psychosis in Four East African Societies. American Anthropologist 68:408–425.

Ehrenberg, A. 2011 Das Unbehagen in der Gesellschaft. Berlin: Suhrkamp.

Ernst, W. 1991 Mad Tales from the Raj: The European Insane in British India, 1800–1858. London: Routledge.

Ernst, W., and T. Mueller, eds. 2010 Transnational Psychiatries: Social and Cultural Histories of Psychiatries in Comparative Perspective, c. 1800–2000. Newcastle: Cambridge Scholars Publishing.

Favret-Saada, J. 1980 Deadly Words: Witchcraft in the Bocage. Cambridge: Cambridge University Press.

Fortune, R. 1932 Sorcerers of Dobu: The Social Anthropology of the Dobu Islanders of the Western Pacific. London: Routledge & Kegan Paul.

Foucault, M. 1967 Madness and Civilization: A History of Insanity in the Age of Reason. London: Tavistock Publications.

———. 1978 The History of Sexuality. Volume I: An Introduction. New York: Pantheon.

Freud, S. 1995 [1913] Totem und Tabu: Einige Übereinstimmungen im Seelenleben der Wilden und der Neurotiker. Frankfurt: Fischer.

Fulford, K. W. M. 1996 Religion and Psychiatry. Extending the Limits of Tolerance. *In* Psychiatry and Religion: Context, Consensus and Controversies. D. Bhugra, ed. Pp. 5–22. London: Routledge.

Fulford, K. W. M., and Z. Sadler 2011 Mapping the Logical Geography of Delusion and Spiritual Experience. *In* Religious and Spiritual Issues in Psychiatric Diagnosis. J. R. Peteet, F. Lu, and W. E. Narrow, eds. Pp. 228–258. Arlington, VA: American Psychiatric Association.

Gaines, A. D., ed. 1992 Ethnopsychiatry: The Cultural Construction of Professional and Folk Psychiatries. Albany: State University of New York Press.

Gilman, S. 1985 Difference and Pathology: Stereotypes of Sexuality, Race, and Madness. Ithaca, NY: Cornell University Press.

Goddard, M. 2011 Out of Place: Madness in the Highlands of Papua New Guinea. New York: Berghahn.

Good, B. J. 1994 Medicine, Rationality, and Experience. Cambridge: Cambridge University Press.

Good, B. J., M. M. J. Fischer, S. S. Willen, and M.-J. DelVecchio Good, eds. 2010 A Reader in Medical Anthropology: Theoretical Trajectories, Emergent Realities. Oxford: Wiley-Blackwell.

Habermas, J. 2005 Zwischen Naturalismus und Religion. Frankfurt: Suhrkamp.

Halliburton, M. 2005 Just Some Spirits: The Erosion of Spirit Possession and the Rise of 'Tension' in South India. Medical Anthropology 24(2):111–144.

Heclo, H., and W. M. McClay, eds. 2003 Religion Returns to the Public Square: Faith and Policy in America. Washington, DC: Woodrow Wilson Center Press.

Heelas, P. 2005 The Spiritual Revolution: Why Religion Is Giving Way to Spirituality. Oxford: Blackwell.

———. 2011 Spiritualities of Life: New Age Romanticism and Consumptive Capitalism. Malden, MA: Wiley-Blackwell.

Hervieu-Léger, D. 2004 Pilger und Konvertiten: Religion in Bewegung. Würzburg: ERGON.

Horwitz, A., and J. Wakefield 2007 The Loss of Sadness: How Psychiatry Transformed Normal Sorrow into Depressive Disorder. Oxford: Oxford University Press.

Howells, W. W. 1948 The Heathens: Primitive Man and His Religions. Garden City, NY: Doubleday.

Huguelet, P., and H. K. Koenig, eds. 2009 Religion and Spirituality in Psychiatry. New York: Cambridge University Press.

Incayawar, M., R. Wintrob, and L. Bouchard, eds. 2009 Psychiatrists and Traditional Healers: Unwitting Partners in Global Mental Health. Chichester: Wiley-Blackwell.

Jadhav, S. 1995 The Ghostbusters of Psychiatry. The Lancet 345(8953):808–810.

———, dir. 2010 The Bloomsbury Cultural Formulation Interview [motion picture]. University College London.

Jenkins, J. H. 2011 Pharmaceutical self: the global shaping of experience in an age of psychopharmacology. Santa Fe, NM: School for Advanced Research Press.

———. 2015 Extraordinary Conditions: Culture and Experience in Mental Illness. Oakland: University of California Press.

Jenkins, J. H., and R. J. Barrett, eds. 2004 Schizophrenia, Culture, and Subjectivity. Cambridge: Cambridge University Press.

Jilek, W. G. 1995 Emil Kraepelin and Comparative Sociocultural Psychiatry. European Archives of Psychiatry and Clinical Neuroscience 245(4-5):231–238.

Jones, J. W. 2004 Religion, Health, and the Psychology of Religion: How the Research on Religion and Health Helps Us Understand Religion. Journal of Religion and Health 43(4):317–328.

Josephson, A. M., and J. R. Peteet 2004 Handbook of Spirituality and Worldview in Clinical Practice. Washington, DC: American Psychiatric.

Kaiser, P. 2007 Religion in der Psychiatrie: Eine (un-)bewußte Verdrängung. Göttingen: Vandenhoek & Ruprecht

Kapur, R. L. 1975 Mental Health Care in Rural India: A Study of Existing Patterns and Their Implications for Future Policy. British Journal of Psychiatry 127:286–93.

Katz, M. M., A. Marsella, K. C. Dube, M. Olatawura, R. Takahashi, Y. Nakane, L. C. Wynne, T. Gift, J. Brennan, N. Sartorius, and A. Jablenksy 1988 On the Expression of Psychosis in Different Cultures: Schizophrenia in an Indian and in a Nigerian Community. Culture, Medicine and Psychiatry 12(3):331–355.

Kendall, L. 2009 The Global Reach of Gods and the Travels of Korean Shamans. *In* Transnational Transcendence: Essays on Religion and Globalization. T. J. Csordas, ed. Pp. 303–327. Berkeley: University of California Press.

Kessler, R., T. B. Ustun, and World Health Organization, eds. 2008 The WHO World Mental Health Surveys: Global Perspectives on the Epidemiology of Mental Disorders. Cambridge: Cambridge University Press.

Kirmayer, L. J. 2004 The Cultural Diversity of Healing: Meaning, Metaphor and Mechanism. British Medical Bulletin 69(1):33–48.

———. 2006 Culture and Psychotherapy in a Creolizing World. Transcultural Psychiatry 43(2):163–168.

———. 2007 Psychotherapy and the Cultural Concept of the Person. Transcultural Psychiatry 44:232–257.

———. 2013 50 Years of Transcultural Psychiatry. Transcultural Psychiatry 50(1):3–5.

Kirmayer, L. J., and H. Minas 2000 The Future of Cultural Psychiatry: An International Perspective. Canadian Journal of Psychiatry 45(5): 438–446.

Kleinman, A. 1977 Depression, Somatization and the 'New Cross-Cultural Psychiatry'. Social Science and Medicine 11(1):3–10.

———. 1980 Patients and Healers in the Context of Culture. Berkeley: University of California Press.

———. 1987 Anthropology and Psychiatry: The Role of Culture in Cross-Cultural Research on Illness. British Journal of Psychiatry 151:447–454.

———. 1988 Rethinking Psychiatry: From Cultural Category to Personal Experience. New York: Free Press.

Kraepelin, E. 2006 [1918] Hundert Jahre Psychiatrie: Ein Beitrag zur Geschichte menschlicher Gesittung. Saarbrücken: Verlag Dr. Müller.

Krause, K. 2006 The Double Face of Subjectivity: A Case Study in a Psychiatric Hospital (Ghana). *In* Multiple Medical Realities: Patients and Healers in Biomedical, Alternative and Traditional Medicine. H. Johanssen and I. Lázár, eds. Pp. 54–71. Oxford: Berghahn.

Kray, C. A. 2002 The Pentecostal Re-Formation of Self: Opting for Orthodoxy in Yucatan. Ethos 29(4):395–429.

Laderman, C., and M. Roseman 1996 The Performance of Healing. New York: Routledge.

Latour, B. 1991 We Have Never Been Modern. Cambridge, MA: Harvard University Press.

———. 2007 Reassembling the Social: An Introduction to Actor Network Theory. Oxford: Oxford University Press.

———. 2010 On the Modern Cult of Factish Gods. Durham, NC: Duke University Press.

Leavey, G. 2004 Identity and Belief within Black Pentecostalims: Spiritual Encounters with Psychiatry. *In* Identity and Health. D. Kelleher and G. Leavey, eds. Pp. 37–58. London: Routledge.

Leckie, J. 2004 Modernity and the Management of Madness in Colonial Fiji. Paideuma 50:251–274.

Lehmann, D. 2004 Religion and Globalization. *In* Religions in the Modern World: Traditions and Transformations. P. Fletcher, H. Kawanami, and D. Smith, eds. Pp. 407–428. London: Routledge.

Lévi-Strauss, C. 1955 The Structural Study of Myth. Journal of American Folklore 68(270):428–444.

Lim, R. 2013 What's New in DSM-5 for Cultural Psychiatry. Psychiatric News. psychnews.psychiatryonline.org/doi/10.1176/appi.pn.2013.10b12.

Littlewood, R. 1990 From Categories to Contexts: A Decade of the 'New Cross-Cultural Psychiatry'. The British Journal of Psychiatry 156(3):308–327.

———. 2000 Psychiatry's Culture. *In* Anthropological Approaches to Psychological Medicine: Crossing Bridges. V. Skultans and J. Cox, eds. Pp. 66–93. London: Jessica Kingsley Publishers.

Littlewood, R., and M. Lipsedge 1985 Culture-Bound Syndromes. *In* Recent Advances in Clinical Psychiatry. K. Granville-Grossman, ed. Pp. 105–142. Edinburgh: Churchill Livingstone.

———. 1997 Aliens and Alienists: Ethnic Minorities and Psychiatry. Hove: Routledge-Brunner.

Littlewood, R., and S. Dein 2013 Did Christianity Lead to Schizophrenia? Psychosis, Psychology and Self-Reference. Transcultural Psychiatry 50(3):397–420.

Lock, M. 2004 Medicalization and the Naturalization of Social Control. *In* Encyclopedia of Medical Anthropology. C. R. Ember and M. Ember, eds. Pp. 116–125. New York: Kluwer Academic/Plenum Publishers.

Luedke, T. J., and H. G. West, eds. 2006 Borders and Healers: Brokering Therapeutic Resources in Southeast Africa. Bloomington, IN: Indiana University Press.

Luhrmann, T. M. 1989 Persuasions of the Witch's Craft: Ritual Magic in Contemporary England. Cambridge, MA: Harvard University Press.

———. 2000 Of Two Minds: The Growing Disorder in American Psychiatry. New York: Knopf.

Mahone, S., and M. Vaughan, eds. 2007 Psychiatry and Empire. Basingstoke: Palgrave Macmillan.

Malinowski, B. 1937 [1927] Sex and Repression in Savage Society. London: Kegan Paul.

Marriott, M. 1976 Hindu Transactions: Diversity without Dualism. *In* Transaction and Meaning: Directions in the Anthropology of Exchange and Symbolic Meaning. B. Kapferer, ed. Pp. 109–142. Philadelphia: ISHI.

Mauss, M. 1985 [1938] A Category of the Human Mind: The Notion of Person; the Notion of Self. *In* The Category of the Person: Anthropology,

Philosophy, History. M. Carrithers, S. Collins, and S. Lukes, eds. Pp. 1–25. Cambridge: Cambridge University Press.

Maxwell, D. 1998. 'Delivered from the Spirit of Poverty?' Pentecostal Discourses of Femininity in Zimbabwe. Journal of Religion in Africa 28(3):278–315.

McCulloch, J. 1995 Colonial Psychiatry and 'the African Mind'. Cambridge: Cambridge University Press.

McDaniel, J. 1989 The Madness of the Saints: Ecstatic Religion in Bengal. Chicago: University of Chicago Press.

Meyer, B. 2002 Commodities and the Power of Prayer: Pentecostalist Attitudes Towards Consumption in Contemporary Ghana. *In* The Anthropology of Globalization. J. X. Inda and R. Rosaldo, eds. Pp. 247–269. New York: Blackwell.

Meyer, B., and P. Pels, eds. 2003 Magic and Modernity: Interfaces between Revelation and Concealment. Stanford, CA: Stanford University Press.

Naraindas, H. 2011 Of Relics, Body Parts and Laser Beams: The German Heilpraktiker and His Ayurvedic Spa. Anthropology & Medicine 18(1):67–86.

Naraindas, H., J. Quack, and W. Sax, eds 2014 Asymmetrical Conversations: Contestations, Circumventions, and the Blurring of Therapeutic Boundaries. Oxford: Berghahn.

Needham, R. 1972 Belief, Language, and Experience. Oxford: Basil Blackwell.

Nichter, M. 1981 Idioms of Distress: Alternatives in the Expression of Psychosocial Distress. A Case Study from South India. Culture, Medicine and Psychiatry 5:379–408.

Nunley, M. 1994 The Mind Doctor's Dharma: On the Social Construction of Hospital Psychiatry in Eastern Uttar Pradesh. San Francisco: University of California.

Pakaslahti, A. 2009 Health-Seeking Behavior for Psychiatric Disorders in North India: An Exploration of Medical Pluralism. *In* Psychiatrists and Traditional Healers: Unwitting Partners in Global Mental Health. M.

Incayawar, R. Wintrob, and L. Bouchard, eds. Pp. 149–166. London: Wiley-Blackwell.

Peteet, J. R., F. G. Lu, and W. E. Narrow 2011 Religious and Spiritual Issues in Psychiatric Diagnosis: A Research Agenda for DSM-V. Arlington, VA: American Psychiatric Association.

Pfeiffer, M. 1994 Transkulturelle Psychiatrie. Stuttgart: Thieme.

Porter, R. 1987 A Social History of Madness: The World through the Eyes of the Insane. London: Weidenfeld & Nicolson.

Prince, M., V. Patel, S. Saxena, M. Maj, J. Maselko, M. R. Phillips, and A. Rahman 2007 No Health without Mental Health. Lancet 370:859–877.

Robbins, J. 2002 My Wife Can't Break Off Part of Her Belief and Give It to Me: Apocalyptic Interrogations of Christian Individualism among the Urapmin of Papua New Guinea. Paideuma 48:189–206.

Rose, N. S. 1996 Inventing Our Selves: Psychology, Power, and Personhood. Cambridge: Cambridge University Press.

———. 2007 The Politics of Life Itself: Biomedicine, Power, and Subjectivity in the Twenty-First Century. Princeton, NJ: Princeton University Press.

Sadowsky, J. 1999 Imperial Bedlam: Institutions of Madness in Colonial Southwest Nigeria. Berkeley: University of California Press.

Sax, W. 2004 Healing Rituals: A Critical Performative Approach. Anthropology & Medicine 11(3):293–306.

———. 2009 God of Justice: Ritual Healing and Social Justice in the Central Himalayas. New York: Oxford University Press.

Sax, W., and J. Weinhold 2010 Rituals of Possession. *In* Ritual Matters: Dynamic Dimensions in Practice. C. Brosius and U. Hüsken, eds. Pp. 236–252. London: Routledge.

Schumaker, J. F., ed. 1992 Religion and Mental Health. Oxford: Oxford University Press.

Scull, A. 1991 Psychiatry and Social Control in the Nineteenth and Twentieth Centuries. History of Psychiatry 2 (6):149–69.

Sébastia, B., ed. 2013 Restoring Mental Health in India. New York: Oxford University Press.

Seligman, C. G. 1929 Temperament, Conflict and Psychosis in a Stone-Age Population. British Journal of Medical Psychology 9:187–202.

Shorter, E. 1997 A History of Psychiatry: From the Era of the Asylum to the Age of Prozac. New York: Wiley.

———. 2009 Before Prozac: The Troubled History of Mood Disorders in Psychiatry. Oxford: Oxford University Press.

Sluhovsky, M. 2007 Believe Not Every Spirit: Possession, Mysticism and Discernment in Early Modern Catholicism. Chicago: University of Chicago Press.

Silverman, J. 1967 Shamans and Acute Schizophrenia. American Anthropologist 69(1):21–31.

Skultans, V. 1997 A Historical Disorder: Neurasthenia and the Testimony of Lives in Latvia. Anthropology & Medicine 4(1):17.

Steinforth, A. S. 2009 Troubled Minds: On the Cultural Construction of Mental Disorder and Normality in Southern Malawi. Frankfurt: Peter Lang.

Strathern, M. 1988 The Gender of the Gift: Problems with Women and Problems with Society in Melanesia. Berkeley: University of California Press.

Styers, R. 2004 Making Magic: Religion, Magic and Science in the Modern World. Oxford: Oxford University Press.

Taylor, C. 1989 Sources of the Self : The Making of the Modern Identity. Cambridge, MA: Harvard University Press.

Vaughan, M. 1991 Curing Their Ills: Colonial Power and African Illness. Stanford, CA: Stanford University Press.

Verhagen, P. J., H. M. Van Praag, J. J. López-Ibor, J. Cox, and D. Moussaoui, eds. 2010 Religion and Psychiatry: Beyond Boundaries. Chichester: Wiley-Blackwell.

Verhagen, P. J., and C. C. H. Cook 2010 Epilogue: Proposal for a World Psychiatric Consensus or Position Statement on Spirituality and Religion in Psychiatry. *In* Religion and Psychiatry: Beyond Boundaries. P. J. Verhagen, H. M. Van Praag, J. J. López-Ibor, J. Cox, and D. Moussaoui, eds. Pp. 615–631. Chichester: Wiley-Blackwell.

Wald, K. D., and A. Calhoun-Brown 2014 Religion and Politics in the United States. Lanham, ML: Rowman & Littlefield.

Whitley, R. 2012 Religious Competence as Cultural Competence. Transcultural Psychiatry 49(2):245–260.

WHO 1973 International Pilot Study of Schizophrenia. Geneva: World Health Organization.

———. 2014a Mental Health: A State of Well-Being. www.who.int/features/factfiles/mental_health/en/

———. 2014b Mental Health Atlas. Geneva: World Health Organization.

Whyte, S. R. 1989 Anthropological Approaches to African Misfortune: From Religion to Medicine. *In* Culture, Experience, and Pluralism: Essays on African Ideas of Illness and Healing. A. Jacobson-Widding and D. Westerlund, eds. Pp. 289–302. Uppsala: Almquist & Wiksell International.

Wilce, J. 2004 Madness, Fear and Control in Bangladesh: Clashing Bodies of Power/Knowledge. Medical Anthropology Quarterly 18(3):357–375.

Wintrob, R. 2009 Overview: Looking Toward the Future of Shared Knowledge and Healing Practices. *In* Psychiatrists and Traditional Healers: Unwitting Partners in Global Mental Health. M. Incayawar, R. Wintrob and L. Bouchard. Pp. 1–12. Chichester: Wiley-Blackwell.

Young, A. 2003 Evolutionary Narratives about Mental Disorders. Anthropology & Medicine 10(2):239–253.

———. 2005 Book Review: Post-Traumatic Stress Disorder: Malady or Myth? Transcultural Psychiatry 42(1):155–157.

———. 2008 A Time to Change Our Minds: Anthropology and Psychiatry in the 21st Century. Culture, Medicine and Psychiatry 32(2):298–300.

# Chapter 1

# The "Seligman Error" and the Origins of Schizophrenia

*Roland Littlewood*

**Introduction**

In 1929 C. G. Seligman, an academic anthropologist and physician, published a paper in the *British Journal of Medical Psychology*, a journal which published work in psychoanalysis and was favorable to social anthropology of a cognitive or psychological bent. Seligman argued that severe mental illness was unknown in early contact New Guinea except in situations of considerable Westernization (Seligman 1929). He was subsequently criticized by both psychiatrists and anthropologists for ignoring psychosis which may be latent but concealed in patterns of spirit possession, ritual performance or other apparently normative social roles—the celebrated "Seligman error."[1] Though apparently a problem of epidemiology, those who have wrestled with it were concerned with detailing the links between society, psychology and psychosis.

Charles Seligman (1873–1940), the son of a Jewish wine merchant, and trained in pathology, had been a member of the Cambridge University Torres Straits expedition of 1898, which is often cited as the start of British ethnographic fieldwork (Herle and Rouse 1998).[2] He became a lecturer in anthropology at the London School of Economics (professor in 1923), where his students included Malinowski and Evans-Pritchard. The paper starts with an apology for using the rather sensational term "stone age population" in his title, yet "I saw a whole fleet of dugouts being constructed with stone adzes." After an account of exceptional and of

---

1  I have not been able to identify the first use of the term. It was certainly current when I was studying anthropology in Oxford in the 1970s. It might have been by my old supervisor, Godfrey Lienhardt, who was an old friend of Brenda Seligman, the widow of C. G. Seligman.
2  Later Seligman famously observed that "field research in anthropology is what the blood of the martyrs is to the church" (Stocking 1996).

limited intelligence in New Guinea, impulsive violence and suggestibility, suicide and epilepsy, Seligman goes on to describe

> brief episodes of transient maniacal excitement among natives who have not been associated with white civilisation [but] no cases of true mental disorder were observed in the villages among natives leading their own normal life . . . [T]he psychoses do not occur except as the stresses set up by white influence, in other words as the consequence of conflict of race, and . . . the result of such conflict is rather to set up a confusional condition than a systematised insanity. [Seligman 1929:195]

He does cite instances of both, but with the latter being apparently due to organic conditions in that the two cases he mentions soon died, and also cites other instances where abnormal behavior was attributed by the individual to an external spirit rather than to himself. Seligman compares these cases with the hysterical dissociations found in early "cargo cults."

Dismissed later in his life for an old-fashioned attachment to racial typologies (e.g., the "Hamitic hypothesis"), Seligman was interested in the origins of technology and he critiqued field ethnography which was not informed by theory; he was marginally influenced by psychoanalysis (employing some of Jung's new ideas) and seems to have been the person who introduced Malinowski to Freud's work (Wallace 1983). During the First World War, he worked with shell shock as did his Torres Straits colleagues Rivers and McDougall (Stocking 1996). Apart from the 1929 paper, he did not write elsewhere on psychiatry in spite of his medical background except for some rather general statements on ethnicity and personality type (Seligman 1932).

Criticism of his paper has come largely from those who favored the idea of the universality and invariance of schizophrenia, but something very like the hypothetical "Seligman error" emerges both in popular anthropology, psychiatry and psychoanalysis, and among the American culture and personality theorists. Both have maintained that it is only in modern Western societies that the antecedents of schizophrenia ("proto-schizophrenia," my term) have emerged as pathological and properly schizophrenic. Both academics and popularizers subscribe to an idea that certain core symptoms of schizophrenia such as certain auditory hallucinations or the loss of subjective agency to external control can be expressed or compensated through social institutions: the most popular choices being shamanism and spirit possession (Silverman 1967). This has often been so extreme that general social anthropologists have been at pains to point out that the average shaman or possessed individual is not conspicuously deviant (Nadel 1946). The countercultural critique, indebted to Jung, Frazer and Eliade, affirms that our patriarchal and capitalist Western civilization has alienated us from a primitive, spiritual ecstatic madness—which has thence emerged with us in frank psychosis, socially misrecognized, stigmatized and segregated. To quote one of the more modest, "modern man no longer knows who he is"; our archaic instincts come to the fore in the modern madman—for schizophrenics are dreaming when awake; the ancient Dionysian rituals involved madness while resistance to them involved even more (Young 1991).

## Was Seligman Right?

Is schizophrenia indeed a modern and European sickness? There are some grounds for thinking so. The idea that Westernization resulted in a higher incidence of schizophrenia was common in the 19th and 20th centuries and was discussed by Kraepelin in 1919. In 1810 Richard Powell had noted insanity was "considerably on the increase," while Andrew Halliday (1828) wrote "we seldom meet with insanity among the savage races of men; not one of our African travellers remark their having seen a single madman" (Hunter and Macalpine 1963:821). We can take these comments with some degree of caution: not only colonial prejudice and Victorian anxieties, but also approximate epidemiology. Imperial psychiatrists in Africa like Tooth and Carothers (as, more recently, Lopez in Brazil, Beaglehole in Hawaii and Dhunjibhoy in India) commented on the infrequency of schizophrenia among communities relatively untouched by colonialism or Westernisation (as reviewed, Torrey 1979, Hopper 2008) but on the high frequency of toxic, confusional or organic symptoms found in apparent schizophrenia (the primary illnesses here may of course have been an infection), but we have to be aware of their fairly prejudicial colonial mind-set. Yet the influential Nigerian psychiatrist Adeoye Lambo (1965) agrees that schizophrenia among non-literate Yoruba is less likely to be associated with systematized chronic delusions and is more confusional, anxious, transitory and affective, while urban Yoruba have the same pattern of schizophrenia as educated modern Europeans.

Anthropologists (who presumably take into account local conceptions of personhood and illness) often draw rather similar conclusions in more detail. Ackerknecht (1943:31, 35) cites some early field studies. Field (1960) argues the association between education and schizophrenia in Ghana is simply that the former makes the illness more visible, but Fortes (Fortes and Mayer 1969), in a different and more administratively remote area, argues rather differently. He carried out his initial fieldwork among the Tallensi of northern Ghana in the 1930s, and then revisited them with his wife, a doctor and medical psychologist, in the 1960s. The Tallensi recognized a chronic pattern called *galuk* characterized by unintelligibility, confused and erratic behavior, an incapacity to carry out normal social and productive tasks, yet clearly distinguished from eccentricity or "other forms of abnormality." Among the local population of around 5,000, Fortes identified in the 1930s only one instance of *galuk* amidst plenty of eccentrics, mentally handicapped and senile individuals. He thinks there were no others and that early death or social concealment by the generally tolerant Tallensi were unlikely. By contrast, among the same villages in the 1960s, with local missionization and some primary education, Fortes and Mayer find 13 cases, and more in neighboring areas: "I had to refuse to see any more" (1969:53). Most of the 13 had previously worked in urban southern Ghana for a period, either as domestic servants or unskilled laborers.

Reviewing data from Ireland and Istria, Murphy (1982) argues high rates of schizophrenia occur in situations of "conflicting or unduly complex demands"; considering the low rates among Tongans and Taiwanese, he speculates that their culture is less individualistic. Devereux (1970) proposes schizophrenia as a Western illness of acculturation and oppression. Communities in the early stages of Westernization are uncommon now, but the World Health Organization's various studies on schizophrenia have found in developing countries a lesser prevalence, better prognosis, shorter episodes and a more affective presentation. Hopper (2007) argues that the relationship of schizophrenia to the acute transient psychoses of the sort commonly described in the third world (the *bouffées délirantes* of Franco-Cuban psychiatry) "remains unsolved" (see also Leff 1981). Working from contemporary Western symptoms, he argues that there has been a shift from bodily to psychological modes of expression: the bodily equivalents of delusions of control are the symptoms of catatonia (waxy flexibility, *mitgehen*, echopraxia and echolalia) more common in developing and rural societies. Jablensky (1987) argues that schizophrenia is more severe and chronic in modernized societies and with industrialization (similarly Wing, Cooper and Sartorius [1976] who favor aspects of social response). Hopper (2008) summarizes the arguments in a recent chapter.

And the historical evidence? Early Babylonian, Egyptian, Hebrew and Indian texts refer to what we may take as insanity: "impulsive, uncontrolled and unreasonable behaviour" (Rosen 1968:32) but not in any systematic way; there is simply a general recognition of irrational behavior along with a demonological explanation. Ideally the term used for this by physicians or other experts in earlier eras should be supplemented by popular lay perceptions (MacDonald 1987), but the early experts did not amplify their diagnoses with the sort of description we need. Without such evidence we cannot easily accept such statements as this by Zilboorg (1941:45) about the classical Greeks: "There were certain mental disturbances, obvious even to the lay person of our day, which continued to remain unrecognised." It appears likely in fact that the Greeks did not clearly distinguish "madness" (μανία, μαινομενous) as psychosis from "delirium" (παράνοια, παράφρονεοντous). The Hippocratic corpus (Hippocrates 1923) often places the two together and uses both to refer to something in the course of a fever. There is no word for, or description of, chronic psychosis here unless this was subsumed into acute madness or delirium, and both Simon (1978) and Evans and colleagues (Evans, McGrath and Kilns 2003) state there is no mention of anything like schizophrenia in Greece, and that μανία (mania) simply connotes "frenzy." Madness in myth, epic and tragedy relies on extremes of passion (Padel 1981), with associated temporary illusions (mistaken perceptions) (Rosen 1968). However, there is an image of chronic madness in tragedy (Padel 1981), and Jeste et al. (1985) argue that there are historical descriptions of something like schizophrenia but that the symptoms have changed over time, while Devereux (1970) confidently identifies an increase during the decline of Rome. Certainly in the later Roman period, Philo recounts a case of a quiet and chronic madman (Rosen 1968) as does Aretaeus (Zilboorg 1941), and Galen and Soranus, in the Christian era, both note that mania occurred without fever (Diethelm 1971); in the first century C.E., Celsus does refer to a "third type" of insanity, characterized by false images or disordered judgment (Jeste et al. 1985), but it was often associated with inappropriate laughter and "foolish amuse[ment]" and thus might correspond to modern mania (Evans, McGrath and Kilns 2003) rather than to schizophrenia.

Like Diethelm, Hunter and Macalpine (1963), in their selection of early modern and modern texts in British psychiatry, easily tag past descriptions with a label of "schizophrenia"; it seems wiser to refer to accounts where we have some more detailed contemporary description of the patients. And here we have a long gap between Hippocrates and Galen and the 17th century English divine and astrologer Richard Napier, who kept modestly detailed records and clinical descriptions of his patients. Napier (or rather his biographer who examined the casebooks statistically) finds a higher-than-expected proportion of young adults among those severely mentally disturbed, an association with villages with a transient population and those with a higher-than-average proportion of both (presumably more religiously observant) Puritans and Catholics (MacDonald 1981). His "most flamboyant and recognisable kinds of insanity" (madness, lunacy and distraction) are comparatively rare and account for five percent of consultations: they are characterized by incoherent speech and unpredictable suicides, by aimless wandering, sudden changes of mood, assaults, self-mutilation and the destruction of others' and their own property. These are all distinguished from melancholia and from what we would now term situational and neurotic complaints. MacDonald notes that it was only later that Locke's emphasis on cognition and perception was to place delusions in madness rather than, as previously, in melancholy (thus suggesting that Napier might have underemphasized the amount of insanity by placing it under melancholia).

Going back to less detailed accounts, the Anglo-Saxon literature mentions instances of chronic insanity such as a four-year history (Clarke 1975), but those recorded are miraculous cures and hence presumably cases with a good prognosis. Cognitive changes are sometimes noted: "his powers of speech, discussion and understanding failed him utterly" (Clarke 1975:42). De Gordon in the 14th century mentions talking to oneself, failure to finish sentences or explain them, meaningless remarks and aimless wandering, affective lability and attempts to grasp the impossible and irrational with poor judgement (Clarke 1975). Clarke describes at length the case of the English king Henry VI: prudish, passive, religiously obsessed and habitually dressed in black; at age 31 he had an illness recalling catatonia, which lasted for six months, plus two relapses, some one and a half years in all.

Clarke (1975) favors such biographical data when we can get it, to avoid the emphasis on the obviously acute and frenzied cases which in the medieval period and later were dealt with by immediate physical restriction rather than observation. By the 16th century chronic madmen (Tom O'Bedlams) were commonly seen around Britain (Clarke 1975). Thomas Willis in his *Soul of Brutes* (1674) said there was no need to give any illustrations but notes their "incongruous notions" (Clarke 1975:294; Hunter and Macalpine 1963); the pattern of severe mental illness was apparently well known. Lunacy (*insania, furor, mania*) now was generally distinguished from *phrenyse*, which occurred only with a fever (Clarke 1975), but there was little psychological description: simply "like a wylde beast" (Hunter and Macalpine 1963:14). By the 19th century, it was common to remark psychological symptoms like "loss of affect" and detachment from surroundings (Hunter and Macalpine 1963), and social and cultural explanations had appeared. In the early 19th century it was recognized that there had been an increase in incidence in Western Europe, especially in the towns rather than the countryside, and especially in England (Hunter and Macalpine 1963), although doubts were raised about selective bias in the statistics. In 1837, rates of insanity were approximately 1 in 1,000 in Europe (in Scotland 1 in 574) as opposed to 1 in 262 in the US in a survey that took some account of bias and data selection.

There is some evidence then that the transition to Western European modernity, both historically and culturally, has been associated with a pattern of psychosis which, compared with its predecessors, is less "affective," less florid and confused, which is associated with lasting cognitive changes such as delusions, and is more chronic with a worse prognosis: in short, something resembling our current idea of schizophrenia. Among the cultural changes that have accompanied this, observers have attributed a variety of not unrelated patterns—"social change" in general, traumatic social change, urbanization, industrialization, modern education, literacy, Christianization, individualism and conscious self-awareness. In the rest of this paper I wish to comment on different "out-related" possibilities as to how "proto-schizophrenia" might have been concealed or compensated in non-Western, non-modern societies (thus leading to the "Seligman error"). The arguments presented here are not mutually exclusive.

**Five Possible "Errors"**

*1. Schizophrenic (or Proto-Schizophrenic) Symptoms are Concealed in Normative Social Institutions such as Shamanism or Spirit Possession*

This we might feel is more probable in psychiatric, rather than in the socially more intensive anthropological, observation. It seems most likely in the acute phase of psychosis, when hallucinations of different types, and responses to hallucinations, abnormal movements, loss of agency and passivity experiences can all be attributed locally to some spirit, which has supplanted the self and agency of the individual. To the external observer, these would be difficult to distinguish from normative possession experiences: unless they are conspicuously deviant—and as I shall argue below, they are perhaps less likely to be channeled in a locally deviant direction if there are available normative models for unusual behavior such as different kinds of spirits. Although possession trance is uncommon in Seligman's original Papuan site, dissociative states and other forms of trance are not.

"By its fruits . . ." concealment in institutional ritual would be less evident in the case of a chronic process, but continued actions and experience alien to local norms might of course still be attributed to a possessing spirit. Laubscher's rather colonial but not unsympathetic account of mental illness among the Tembu of South Africa in 1937 described the local experience of *ukuthwasa*: when the River People spirits call a Tembu he becomes listless and aimless, loses weight and experiences aches and pains and bad dreams. Suddenly he runs for the river and jumps in; under the water he learns divination and healing; and emerging some ten days later he begins to practice as a healer. The local diviners, the *isanuses*, tell Laubscher that *ukuthwasa* is the call for a training with the River People which only they have undergone. Other local healers (who are regarded as charlatans both by Laubscher and the *isanuses*) also claim the same experience. Patients in the local psychiatric hospital claim too to have undergone *ukuthwasa* and describe the underwater world. The local population says many people have jumped in and drowned. The Tembu, says Laubscher the psychiatrist, recognize all types of auditory hallucinations as *ukuthwasa* but distinguish them from the toxic psychoses of delirium or fever, and use this single descriptive category to describe both the visions of the seer and the experiences of what the psychiatrists would term mental illness. A continued illness is then the residual failure to successfully achieve full training or else to reject it. Similarly, chronic insanity in South America may be regarded as the failure to respond to a shamanic call, while Field (1960) describes depression in Ghana as obscured by ritual self-accusations of witchcraft. The WHO's Present State Examination allows for something like this in its categories of subcultural delusions and hallucinations, which may be psychiatrically abnormal but are incorporated into locally recognized experiences (Wing, Cooper and Sartorius 1976).

## 2. Schizophrenia in Non-Western, Non-Modern Societies is Transient

We have seen that there is some contemporary evidence for this. If schizophrenia (or proto-schizophrenia) is short-lived, then not only is it likely to be missed by the psychiatric observer not being on site at the time, but if the local recognition of it places it in some domain of unsought spirit possession, then again it is less likely to be reported to the observer when resolved subsequently and, if it is, it may be difficult to distinguish it in the report from "everyday" (dissociative) spirit possession. Thus, although less likely in the case of schizophrenia, as a pattern, it falls into a general area of other transient alterations of the normal sensorium: altered states of consciousness in psychoactive drug use and hypnogogic hallucinations, acute psychotic reactions and perhaps the phasic alterations of manic depressive illness and the fevers often locally ascribed to the prodromal call to shamanism, vision quest or "crisis cult" inspiration. And when the alteration ceases, the experiences are "worked up" by the protagonist and others in terms of the local social logic, experience and actions associated with such episodes, which may be then "imitated" by the community and the original (pathological?) instance in retrospect becomes less idiosyncratic (Littlewood 1993). Thus, La Barre gives the example of Evara of the Papua "*Vaihala* madness" as spreading "a stylised epilepsy in his group apparently genuine in him originally" (1972:316).[3]

---

3 A nice example, but La Barre's source (Williams 1934) merely says that

An example of this from my own fieldwork is the leader of a religious community in Trinidad, the Earth People, who experienced visions and a sense of cosmic power after childbirth in a remote and abandoned village: visions and authority which later, after they ended, were consolidated by discussions within the family and through proselytization, which eventually gave rise to a whole community based on her interpretation of these experiences (Littlewood 1993). When interviewed by me she was no longer psychiatrically abnormal[4] and her original cosmological interpretation of her psychotic experiences had become normative doctrine for the whole group. Although she had probably been hypomanic, if we allow proto-schizophrenia experiences a similar transient form, then we may conclude they too may pass into subsequently accepted beliefs and actions—and thus be less salient as abnormality. As Ohlmarks (1939) remarked, an institution may originate in pathological individual experience which becomes "structured" through the response of others, a possibility suggested by Bogoras' original description of a Chuckchee shaman who was periodically insane (when she was restrained physically) while practicing successfully during her lucid periods.

### 3. *Proto-Schizophrenia Only Becomes Schizophrenia through Social Response*

Firth (1973), without citing specific instances, maintains that non-industrial societies are more tolerant of the symbolizations of mental illness

---

Evara had had "ecstatic seizures" for some time before the movement began. For a more critical account of the Western Pacific imitation of epilepsy, see Hoskins (1967). The Amerindian Shakers institutionalized a form of shaking originally "spontaneous" (Barnett 1953), while a more bizarre example of the "imitation of madness" (Littlewood 1993) is among the Canadian Doukhobors for whom delirium and intoxication in the elders were oracular and thence imitable communications (Hawthorne 1955).

4   Though diagnosed as schizophrenic by the local psychiatrists (I consulted her hospital notes), when I met her she only scored minor neurotic symptoms on the Present State Examination (Wing, Cooper and Sartorius 1976), but retrospectively for the time of her inspiration her experiences yielded the category M+ on the PSE, equivalent to the manic phase of bipolar disorder. She had a diffusely enlarged thyroid, a high resting pulse, heat intolerance and subsequently died of cardiac failure. I think it is likely that she had Graves' disease with thyrotoxic episodes at the time of her pregnancies and visions.

and are more likely to enter into a successful dialogue with them. And similar ideas occur in the modern Hearing Voices Network. Weston La Barre's book *The Ghost Dance* (La Barre 1972) took its title from the Plains Indians' movement of 1890 in which various tribes joined together under the inspiration of Wovoka following the loss of their hunting territories to the Europeans, the virtual disappearance of the once ubiquitous buffalo and a succession of crushing military defeats, new and fatal diseases and devastating droughts. On his recovery from an illness, in the course of which an eclipse of the sun had occurred, Wovoka preached a new ritual dance, through the performance of which a fresh skin would spread over the earth, bearing pasture and herds, and covering up the whites and their works. La Barre offers the Ghost Dance as the paradigm for all religions, indeed for all novel collective actions.

Religious innovators, he suggests, are culture healers with personal visions which are essentially mental illnesses,[5] asocial and idiosyncratic; their "crisis cults" are personal strategies for dealing with anxiety in times of disaster, which can then serve for other individuals, and thus they generate all forms of social change. "Culture is folie à N . . . the only difference between folie and culture is quantitative"—but "the magnitude of the social impact is not an acceptable psychiatric criterion for psychosis [for the] genius is a psycho-social phenomenon as a shaman-messiah only if and when he is dynamically relevant to and functioning in his proper socio-cultural context" (La Barre 1972:343, 317, 273, 351). Similarly, the sociologist Bryan Wilson (1975) observes, "If a man runs naked down the street proclaiming that he alone can save others from impending doom, and if he immediately wins a following, then he is a charismatic leader: a social relationship has come into being. If he does not win a

---

5 Cf. Erikson (1965). It may be objected that I am concentrating here on two figures, La Barre and Devereux, who are relatively marginal to contemporary psychological anthropology. While their particular use of the idioms of psychoanalysis is perhaps idiosyncratic, they do seem to face the question straight on, unlike their Culture and Personality colleagues, Benedict and Kluckhohn, who side-stepped the topic of frank insanity and preferred to talk only of "internal conflicts." But perhaps the only difference is whether one understands these internal conflicts (proto-schizophrenia?) as psychotic or not: in spite of his terminology La Barre does indeed come close to seeing them merely as subjective anxiety.

following, then he is simply a lunatic." To an extent, La Barre sees the origins of proto-schizophrenia as extra-social, an autonomous domain of arbitrary nature which may at times gel with society. However, he defines this domain on psychodynamic grounds alone, identified and perceived backwards from its cultural products, with the result that Plato becomes "a Greek ghost dance[r] . . . a covert paranoid schizophrenic" (La Barre 1972:541). Henry Murphy takes this argument further to suggest that times out of joint ("crises") actually generate psychopathological solutions: "Delusions may occur in times of increased stress as if, in reaction to changing conditions, the culture does call on individual members to sacrifice their mental health by the development of individual delusions which relieve communal anxieties" (Murphy 1967); similarly Erik Erikson argues that leaders are psychological healers who have a "grim willingness to do the dirty work of their ages" (Erikson 1965:317). But these two take us into the hypothetical origin of psychosis rather than its obfuscation (see argument 5).

Georges Devereux, a psychoanalytical anthropologist like La Barre, suggests similarly that the sickness is already located in the prophetic moment; the prophet takes authority when the usual adaptations to stress are inadequate, and society itself is in a "schizophrenic-like disorientation" with individuals engaging in "catastrophic behaviour." The solution adopted is irrational and leads to a vicious circle in which the crisis gets increasingly out of control (Devereux 1955). He proposes schizophrenia as a *psychose ethnique*, a product of violent processes of acculturation and oppression (Devereux 1970) and identifies it as causal psychological detachment and fragmented or over-specialized Western lives (among other factors).

While all the above schemata presume a shamanic or similar role as approximately constant and available through various crises, Jane Murphy suggests that as Inuit shamanism declined as a political institution, increasingly marginal and mentally ill individuals came to aspire to it (Murphy 1964).

## 4. The Recognition of Schizophrenia Requires a Modern Western Psychological Backdrop

The idea of the modern self famously provided by Geertz (1983) is one which is hardly universal: a "bounded, unique, more or less integrated motivational and cognitive universe, a dynamic centre of awareness, emotion, judgement and action organised into a distinctive whole and set contrastively both against other such wholes and against a social and natural background." Fabrega has argued that the "first rank symptoms" of schizophrenia, taken in modern comparative psychiatry as an accurate manifestation of unequivocal schizophrenia, really necessitate such "basic Western assumptions about human action and social reality," particularly cultural conventions of the autonomous self (Fabrega 1982:56). He cites such conventions that persons are independent beings whose minds and bodies are separated from each other and function autonomously; that under ordinary conditions external influences do not affect an individual; that thoughts are recurring inner happenings that the self "has"; that thoughts and feelings are rather different things but that both are silent and private; that one's body is independent of what one feels or thinks and that body and feelings have a purely naturalistic basis and cannot be modified by external ultra-human agents (Fabrega 1982). Barrett (2004), finding the Iban of Borneo have difficulty understanding his questions about two first-rank symptoms, thought insertion and thought broadcasting, argues similarly. His three Iban individuals (contrasted with 39 European Australians in a matched psychotic sample) who experience these symptoms are all converts to Christianity. He suggests an association with education and reading, and a familiarity with the idea of an omniscient God who can tell what is in one's mind (but equal numbers of Iban and Australians experienced auditory hallucinations). Traditional Iban notions of thinking, he proposes, are much more embodied, tied closely to emotion, will and desire: their word for "thought" also denotes "speech." This explanation again shades into the fifth argument.

## 5. The Actual Occurrence of Schizophrenia Requires a Modern Western Psychological Backdrop

Sass (2004), following the work of the phenomenologist Wolfgang Blankenburg, proposes that psychological hyper-reflexivity is significant for fully developed schizophrenia: reflective self-consciousness and other patterns in which the individual comes to focus on itself and on features of its own functioning, associated with a loss of the usual taken-for-granted experience of the local world (what, following Blankenburg, he terms a "loss of self evidence" [2004:305–307], akin to the well-known "delusional mood" of schizophrenia in which the environment is no longer normal for something odd is going on). The initially tacit, including the processes of personal psychological functioning, now becomes the focus of awareness: "a focused, introspective awareness that de-realises sensations by detaching them from the unnoticed background whilst simultaneously subjecting these sensations to processes of externalisation and reification" (Sass 2004:312–313). Aspects of the self are experienced as akin to external objects as the tacit becomes forced, artificial and awkward, and to be examined. Reflecting on this only further distances the person from any sense of naturalness or capacity for spontaneous action, thus exacerbating self-alienation (Sass 2004). Living with this destabilizing cognitive slippage and the loss of the tacit is made worse, says Sass, by those (modern) societies which encourage the same tendencies, in which everybody increasingly lives in a less stable external world and is plunged into idiosyncratic internalized experience, into a set of fragmented pluralistic alternatives in which the act of choice itself becomes problematic and in which the individual self is increasingly restricted in that its processes, indeed it itself, become an object for scrutiny. Sass describes this as "a shift from extraverted traditional societies in which emotional life, organised through myth and ritual, is at the centre to the more introverted modern societies in which intellectual processes are far more dominant" (Sass 2004), to, as we might say, the triumph of psychology as the dominant mode of personal being. Simon Dein and myself have argued (Littlewood and Dein 2013) that this "excessive" reflexive self-consciousness in part originated with Christianity and Christian conversion, and, reinforced by the Reformation and the development of popular everyday secular psychology, has grown in the modern era and is a concomitant of "Westernization" (modernization, psychological internalization) in non-Western societies.

In a neuro-philosophical paper, Kircher and Leube (2003) propose that our first level of consciousness (pre-reflexive consciousness) comprises primary experiences which are tacit and "transparent" in that while the brain constructs our reality the mechanism of this construction is not re-presented in it, thus resulting in naïve realism—the assumption that the content of consciousness has a direct contact to the immediate environment. If we then reflect on primary experiences, the content enters introspective consciousness (level two). Primary self-experiences include self-agency (as well as self-coherence, self-affectivity and autobiographical memory)—the sense that one is the author of one's actions. Life requires a balance between anticipated action planning and control, and proprioceptive feedback: failure leads to incorrect attribution of events to the self, as in schizophrenia where self-monitoring fails. One might speculate that excessive introspective self-consciousness leads to an objectification of experience in level two, with neglect of proprioception leading to a failure in maintaining this balance. Lienhardt (1961) described how in the 1950s pagan Dinkas' everyday emotions and memories were not experienced as subjective but as put into the person through other people and events in the environment: a memory is something external still acting on one (Kircher and Leube's "naïve realism"). The dismantling of such an indigenous psychology makes the "thought insertion" and "made affects" of proto-schizophrenia more problematic and abnormal, as experiences are no longer shared or intelligible to one's fellows: and thus yielding a social response accentuating schizophrenia (as Sass proposes).

## Conclusion

If most of my critical sources are relatively old, this is because the debate has largely been forgotten with the decline of Culture and Personality social anthropology, whose psychoanalytical underpinnings emphasized individual psychology and personality as the intermediate variable between culture and mental illness. Wary of labeling whole societies as pathological we are now reluctant to seek within a society those psychological antecedents which may develop as schizophrenia. Anti-racism and a functionalist emphasis on intensive fieldwork alike have normalized thought and action which once struck the European as bizarre or pathological. At the same time, anthropology, unhappy with the very idiom of pathology, has relinquished to psychiatry the task of defining abnormality. Our current position recalls that of the medical historian Erwin Ackerknecht who in 1943, confident that he could distinguish pathology from culture, criticized Georges Devereux for

the labelling of [social] phenomena with psychiatric diagnosis . . . The custom of covering moral judgements with a pseudoscientific psychopathological nomenclature is no advance at all and is equally bad for both moral and science . . . When religion is but "organised schizophrenia" [Devereux's expression], then there is no room or necessity for history, sociology, etc. God's earth was, and is, but a gigantic state hospital and pathography becomes the unique and universal science. [Ackerknecht 1943][6]

Ackerknecht's solution was to firmly separate the local (emic) perception of normal/abnormal from the medical (etic) perception of the same, thus yielding a possible fourfold classification of illness and disease. To an extent, this recalls the distinction between our naturalistic (scientific) and personalistic (humane) models (Littlewood 1993). Whether such a heuristic (and implicitly relativist) distinction will survive current attempts like those of Sass to edge in from each end in a sort of neuro-sociology is yet to be seen,[7] and also whether this will prove more useful than those of the Culture and Personality theorists who attempted the same. Seligman's "error"—if such it was—opens up to us again a general program for research on society and psychopathology, in which the limitations relativism has (correctly) placed upon us will themselves be incorporated into a more universalized schema.

**Acknowledgements**

This paper was presented as a plenary address to the "3rd World Congress of Cultural Psychiatry" at Queen Mary College, London, 2012. Some of the argument and material has appeared in both a previous paper (Littlewood and Dein 2013) and a book (Littlewood 1993).

**References**

Ackerknecht, E. H. 1943 Psychopathology, Primitive Medicine and Primitive Culture. Bulletin of the History of Medicine 14:30–68.

---

6 Devereux reposted by criticising Ackerknecht for "disregarding the existence of societies so 'sick' that in order to adjust to them, one has to be very sick indeed . . . There exist societies so enmeshed in a vicious circle that everything they do to save themselves only causes them to sink deeper into the quicksand" (Devereux 1956).

7 With less functionalist "steady state" theorizations now, we are more prepared perhaps to consider some "societies" as pathological or "failed" reflections (or victims) of others in our tighter, more globalized—and less relativist—world. We might note that Devereux' and La Barre's instances come particularly from colonized minority groups.

Barnett, H. G. 1953 Innovation: The Basis of Culture Change. New York: McGraw-Hill.

Barrett, R. J. 2004 Kurt Schneider in Borneo: Do First Rank Symptoms Apply to the Iban? *In* Schizophrenia, Culture and Subjectivity. J. H. Jenkins and R. J. Barrett, eds. Pp. 87–109. Cambridge: Cambridge University Press.

Clarke, B. 1975 Mental Disorder in Earlier Britain. Cardiff: University of Wales Press.

Devereux, G. 1955 Charismatic Leadership and Crisis. *In* Psychoanalysis and the Social Sciences. G. Roheim, ed. Pp. 145–157. New York: International Universities Press.

———. 1956 Normal and Abnormal: The Key Problem in Psychiatric Anthropology. *In* Some Uses of Anthropology, Theoretical and Applied. J. Casagrande and T. Gladwin, eds. Pp. 23–48. Washington, DC: Anthropological Society.

———. 1970 Essais d'ethnopsychiatrie générale. Paris: Gallimard.

Diethelm, O. 1971 Medical Dissertations of Psychiatric Illness Printed before 1750. Basel: Karger.

Erikson, E. H. 1965 Childhood and Society. Harmondsworth: Penguin.

Evans, R., J. McGrath, and R. Kilns 2003 Searching for Schizophrenia in Ancient Greek and Roman Literature: A Systematic Review. Acta Psychiatrica Scandinavica 107:323–330.

Fabrega, H. 1982 Culture and Psychiatric Illness. *In* Cultural Conceptions of Mental Health and Therapy. A. J. Marsella and G. M. White, eds. Pp. 39–68. Dordrecht: Reidel.

Field, M. 1960 Search for Security: An Ethno-Psychiatric Study of Rural Ghana. London: Faber and Faber.

Firth, R. 1973 Symbols, Public and Private. London: Allen and Unwin.

Fortes, M., and D. Y. Mayer 1969 Psychosis and Social Change among the Tallensi of Northern Ghana. *In* Psychiatry in a Changing Society. S. H. Foulkes and G. S. Prince, eds. Pp. 33–74. London: Tavistock.

Geertz, C. 1983 Local Knowledge. New York: Basic Books.

Hawthorne, H. 1955 The Doukhobors of British Columbia. London: Dent.

Herle, A., and S. Rouse 1998 Cambridge and the Torres Strait: Centenary Essays on the 1898 Expedition. Cambridge: Cambridge University Press.

Hippocrates 1923 The Sacred Disease. Cambridge, MA: Harvard University Press.

Hopper, K. 2007 [1987] Recovery from Schizophrenia: An International Perspective. A Report from the WHO Collaborative Project, the International Study of Schizophrenia. Oxford: Oxford University Press.

———. 2008 Outcomes Elsewhere: Course of Psychosis in 'Other Cultures'. *In* Society and Psychosis. C. Morgan, K. McKenzie, and P. Fearon, eds. Pp. 198–216. Cambridge: Cambridge University Press.

Hunter, R., and I. Macalpine 1963 Three Hundred Years of Psychiatry. London: Oxford University Press.

Jablensky, A. 1987 Multicultural Studies and the Nature of Schizophrenia: A Review. Journal of the Royal Society of Medicine 80:162–167.

Jeste, D. V., R. Del Carmen, J. R. Lohr, and R. J. Wyatt 1985 Did Schizophrenia Exist before the 18th Century? Comprehensive Psychiatry 26:493–503.

Kircher, T. T. J., and D. T. Leube 2003 Self-Consciousness, Self-Agency, and Schizophrenia. Consciousness and Cognition 12:656–669.

La Barre, W. 1972 The Ghost Dance: Origins of Religion. London: Allen and Unwin.

Lambo, T. A. 1965 Schizophrenia and Borderline States. *In* Transcultural Psychiatry. A. V. S. de Reuck and R. Porter, eds. Pp. 62–75. London: Churchill.

Leff, J. 1981 Psychiatry around the Globe. New York: Dekker.

Lienhardt, G. 1961 Divinity and Experience. Oxford: Clarendon Press.

Littlewood, R. 1993 Pathology and Identity: The Work of Mother Earth in Trinidad. Cambridge: Cambridge University Press.

Littlewood, R., and S. Dein 2013 Did Christianity Cause Schizophrenia? Transcultural Psychiatry 50:397–420.

MacDonald, M. 1981 Mystical Bedlam: Madness, Anxiety and Healing in Seventeenth Century England. Cambridge: Cambridge University Press.

———. 1987 Madness, Suicide and the Computer. *In* Problems and Methods in the History of Medicine. R. Porter and A. Wear, eds. Pp. 207–229. London: Croom Helm.

Murphy, H. B. M. 1967 Cultural Aspects of the Delusion. Studium Generale 2:684–692.

———. 1982 Comparative Psychiatry: The International and Intercultural Distribution of Mental Illness. Berlin: Springer.

Murphy, J. 1964 Psychotherapeutic Aspects of Shamanism on St. Lawrence Island, Alaska. *In* Magic, Faith and Healing. A. Kiev, ed. Pp. 61–69. New York: Free Press.

Nadel, S. F. 1946 A Study of Shamanism in the Nuba Mountains. Journal of the Royal Anthropological Institute 86:25–37.

Ohlmarks, C. A. 1939 Studien zum Problem des Shamanismus. Lund: Gleerup.

Padel, R. 1981 Madness in Fifth-Century (B.C.) Athenian Tragedy. *In* Indigenous Psychologies. P. Heelas and A. Lock, eds. Pp. 105–131. London: Academic Press.

Rosen, G. 1968 Madness in Society. London: Routledge and Kegan Paul.

Sass, L. 2004 'Negative Symptoms', Commonsense and Cultural Disembedding in the Modern Age. *In* Schizophrenia, Culture and Subjectivity. J. H. Jenkins and R. J. Barrett, eds. Pp. 303–328. Cambridge: Cambridge University Press.

Seligman, C. G. 1929 Temperament, Conflict and Psychosis in a Stone-Age Population. British Journal of Medical Psychology 9:187–202.

———. 1932 Anthropological Perspectives and Psychological Theory. Journal of the Royal Anthropological Institute 62:193–228.

Sharp, P. T. 1990 The Searching Sun: The Lyeime Movement—Crisis, Tragic Events and folie à deux in the Papua New Guinea Highlands. Transcultural Psychiatric Research Review 27:225–227.

Silverman, J. 1967 Shamans and Acute Schizophrenia. American Anthropologist 69(1):21–31.

Simon, B. 1978 Mind and Madness in Ancient Greece. Ithaca: Cornell University Press.

Stocking, G. 1996 After Tylor: British Social Anthropology 1888–1951. London: Athlone.

Torrey, E. F. 1979 Schizophrenia and Civilization. New York: Aronson.

Wallace, E. R. 1983 Freud and Anthropology: A History and a Reappraisal. New York: International Universities Press.

Williams, F. E. 1934 The Vaihala Madness in Retrospect. *In* Essays Presented to C. G. Seligman. E. E. Evans-Pritchard, ed. Pp. 369–380. London: Kegan Paul.

Wilson, B. 1975 Noble Savages: The Primitive Origins of Charisma and Its Contemporary Survival. Berkeley: University of California Press.

Wing, J., J. E. Cooper, and N. Sartorius 1976 Measurement and Classification of Psychiatric Symptoms. Cambridge: Cambridge University Press.

Young, D. 1991 Origins of the Sacred: The Ecstasies of Love and War. London: Abacus.

Zilboorg, G. 1941 A History of Medical Psychology. New York: Norton.

## Chapter 2

## Return of the Religious: Good Shamanism and Bad Exorcism

*Andreas Heinz and Anne Pankow*

**Introduction**

In recent years, several articles and conferences have focused on the spiritual needs of patients, particularly in the mental health care system. On the one hand, such discussions focused on questions of how to cope with long-term disorders, the limits of medical technologies and the creation of personally meaningful narratives about personal experiences; on the other hand, they noticed a peculiar absence of professional interest in the spiritual needs of patients (Mönter 2007). What appears to be just another discussion on therapeutic "blind spots" in the mental health care system, however, has far deeper and more profound implications: psychiatry and psychosocial medicine is constantly ridden by questions regarding the legitimacy of standard medical approaches towards human suffering in the presence of competing explanatory models and professionally organized psychosocial systems such as traditional religions, an ever-widening market of new age healing and critical reflections on the fundamental assumptions and "ideological building blocks" of modern psychiatry and psychotherapy. Such discussions are contextualized by a new series of struggles between religious groups and scientific academia, which range from discussions between Creationists and Darwinists to phenomena such as a conference in Graz, Austria, in 2007, which addressed "Religiosity in Psychiatry and Psychotherapy" (www.rpp2007.org) and invited both traditional Catholic exorcists as well as healers active in "conversion therapy," who aim to help homosexuals unhappy with their sexual orientation to alter their sexual preferences. Such phenomena may not only indicate a "return of the uncanny" with respect to a religious interpretation of psychotic symptoms, which had dominated Central European approaches towards "madness" for centuries, but may also have far deeper implications with respect to the construction of mental disorders. As we will point out, psychotic experience had long been compared to more "primitive" and hence more fundamental religious or magical experiences. Modern day romanticism towards such presumably unspoiled and "pure" spiritual experiences may just represent the flipside of a fundamental construction and denigration of the "otherness" of patients suffering from mental disorders, which compared them with colonized people and subjected them to similar forms of social exclusion and extermination (Heinz 1998). To elucidate these aspects of religious practices and beliefs and their impact on subjects with "extraordinary experiences," we will discuss fundamental aspects of the construction of traditional psychiatric nosologies, describe the role that colonial and social hierarchies played in shaping the modern understanding of mental disorders, discuss anti-colonial and anti-psychiatric ideas that questioned such hierarchical ideas about mental health and "normal development" and finally, try to describe the complex space occupied by modern discourses on "spirituality" and religious values in psychiatry.

## Degeneration and Evolution: A Secularization of Religious Concepts to Explain Mental Disorders

At the beginning of the 19th century, "degeneration" was the dominant paradigm used to describe human development: God created man in a perfect state, and subsequent developments led to his downfall and degeneration, which—as some authors suggested—is less prominent in Europeans or Caucasians compared to "Negros" and "Mongoloids" (Heinz 1998). However, degeneration was not limited to populations or "races"—it was a constant threat within a given group of people and was supposed to result from rather small mistakes and indulgences such as excessive alcohol consumption, unruly behavior or "greed" evoked by inappropriate socialist ideas; it was thought to increase with each successive generation. Morel, who articulated one of the leading theories on degeneration in mental disorders, suggested that minor misdemeanors can result in the first signs of degeneration, and that such degenerative traits are heritable and increase in severity in each following generation until finally the whole family dies out due to severe debility or cretinism (Morel 1857).

An example from literature is the famous novel Buddenbrooks by Thomas Mann, which describes the successive downfall of an originally powerful Hanseatic family. Such fantasies of successive degeneration may have

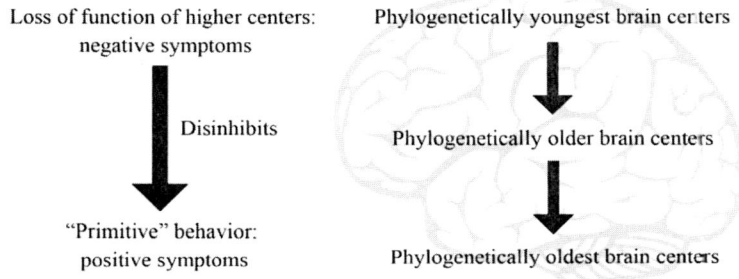

*Figure 1: Hypothesized process of "degeneration." The loss of functions of evolutionary higher brain areas is supposed to manifest as negative symptoms and the disinhibition of evolutionarily older brain areas results in positive symptoms. This model reflects a strict top-down brain hierarchy inspired by social hierarchies and lacks any "bottom-up" or collateral control mechanisms.*

been strongly inspired by the experience of syphilis: here sexual "liberty" leads to a disease and, via intrauterine infection, the fetus can also display "degenerative" traits. Fantasies about the damaging consequences of social libertinage were even stronger given that it was not known until the early 20th century that syphilis is caused by a spirochete, which can also affect a fetus in the uterus. Before this discovery, affection of the offspring was ascribed to the threatening and powerful process of "degeneration," which was used to explain all evils of modern industrialized societies, alcoholism, poverty, social conflicts and diseases spreading in the heavily populated inner cities.

However, concepts of degeneration were hard to reconcile with the modern concept of evolution. If mankind indeed was not created by a divine act in a perfect state, but rather developed from "primitive" roots to its modern day presence, the concept of degeneration would have to be abandoned altogether. Nevertheless, it survived—it seems to have been too powerful an explanatory model, and its impressive capacity to neglect social problems and to ascribe them to individual misdemeanor made it a primary candidate to explain socially unwanted behavior, from criminal felonies to "madness." Indeed, it was suggested that mental disorders or other unruly behaviors reflect a degenerative process that turns "evolution" around: the more severe a mental disorder is, the deeper the degeneration or "regression" to a more primitive evolutionary level. Such speculations may not have caught the attention of medical doctors or the wider public if it had not been for Haeckel's concept of an ontogeny recapitulating phylogeny: Haeckel suggested that evolution is recapitulated in individual development. Indeed, the human embryo at a certain stage resembles a fish rather than a human being; however, modern day biology has criticized this approach and suggested that similarities are limited to intrauterine development (Czihak 1981). Nevertheless, Haeckel's ideas ignited a fury of comparisons between "primitive" levels of human development. Children were a prime example of immature mankind; they have to be guided and educated to become full members of society and to be capable of rational thinking. The same status was attributed to women and to the assumed phylogenetic precursors of modern mankind. However, in the absence of "ice age" man in the world of the 19th century, the populations subjected to colonialism worldwide were taken as a surrogate. This of course meant that their own development throughout the millennia since the ice age was simply denied, just like pre-colonial encounters including mass slavery in Africa, the transatlantic slave trade or the extinction of Native Americans were ignored in the great "evolutionary narratives" of the late 19th and early 20th century. From neurobiology to psychoanalysis it was believed that modern Western mankind, which was limited to "white men," represented the peak of human development, while children, women, subjects suffering from mental disorders and colonized people were all supposed to represent more primitive stages of development (Heinz 1998). While details of the narratives of the alleged evolutionary development from primitive man to modern mankind differed and were often the topic of fierce debates, one main idea characterized all these constructions: there is a unilinear development from primitiveness to modernity, and everybody deviating from the narrow rules of Western adult behavior does so because this evolutionary peak has either never been reached or was lost within mental disorders. A concept of degeneration remained thus at the core of the modern understanding of man; its religious roots are barely disguised in the new, scientific construction of "evolution." Within this framework, moral judgments and denigration of the more "primitive" people reign supreme.

However, placing mentally disordered subjects, particularly psychotic patients, at the bottom of the evolutionary ladder right next to "primitive," colonized people meant that they could easily be subjected to the same aggressive approach. Indeed, "race wars" to exterminate whole nations of Africans were fought in the German colonies: concentration camps were imported into the then German colony of Southwest Africa from British South Africa and used to deliberately exterminate rebellious nations such as the Herero and Nama, before such techniques were imported to Europe in World War II. Also, regulations against "interracial" marriages were developed in the German colonies before similar laws were put into effect in Nazi Germany, and compulsory sterilization laws were enacted not only against mentally disordered patients suffering from presumably heritable diseases but also against the so-called Rhineland Bastards, the black German children of French soldiers who occupied the *Ruhrgebiet* following World War I. The extermination of psychiatric patients during Nazi Germany, promoted and applauded by German psychiatrists but denied when exposed to the public, also resembles the deliberate extermination and official denials thereof in the genocide of the Herero and Nama in colonial Germany (Heinz 1998; Olusoga and Erichsen 2010). Several colonial officers who learned the "art" of genocide in the African colonies later formed right-wing military units (*Freikorps*) that murdered rebellious workers and formed the core of the latter Nazi party, including prominent figures such as Ritter von Epp (Olusoga and Erichsen 2010). Examples of such comparisons between "primitive" people and psychotic patients can be found in a multitude of psychiatric articles and theories. To quote just two: when constructing the new disease entity of "schizophrenia," Bleuler was inspired by Freud and suggested that any modern man is capable of rational thinking, while psychotic patients just like "the Negro" [*sic*] would only be able to indulge in wishful thinking, utterly unable to take reality into consideration. Carothers, the leading British colonial psychiatrist, suggested as late as the 1950s that Africans resemble Europeans whose frontal lobe had willfully been damaged (through, e.g., lobotomy) (McCulloch 1995).

## Alternative Narratives: A Multitude of Languages and Cultural Patterns and the Romantic Craving for the "Other"

With the downfall of Nazi Germany, public discussions of death camps, compulsory sterilization, mass murder of psychiatric patients and previously prevalent eugenic theories about the alleged superiority of the "white race" and its right to rule over different groups of supposedly inferior people were subject to public debate. In anthropology, social theories gained momentum that described the semantic organization of explanatory models in different cultures and compared them rather than ranking them in a unilineal way (Evans-Pritchard 1937; Lévi-Strauss 1962). Within psychiatry and psychoanalysis, it was individuals such as Wilhelm Reich (1973) or the psychoanalyst Erik Erikson (1965) who demanded respect for different human cultures, denied that "primitive" cultures function at a "pre-logic" or "irrational" level and even questioned the concept of "primitivity" itself. In the wake of the 1960s and 1970s a variety of social movements, ranging from the civil rights movement in the US to the student rebellion and feminist groups, questioned the social hierarchies embedded in the evolutionary construction of human development and questioned the social exclusion of minorities and psychiatric patients. However, reform of psychiatric institutions only went so far, and slowed down considerably in the 1980s and 1990s, with large clinics being reduced in size in countries like Italy or Germany or even closed altogether, without individuals suffering from mental problems being fully included in society.

On the other hand, liberated from the stigma of "primitive," "inferior" and "to be exterminated," the "pure," "unspoiled" or "original" (i.e., pre-Western and pre-capitalist) approaches to society and nature gained increasing popularity. While in some cases this took the form of an intellectual criticism of the standards, rules and regulations of modern scientific groups (Kuhn 1962; Feyerabend 1975), there was also an ever-increasing interest in the "easy way" to a "natural" spirituality.

## The Return of the Religious: Good Shamanism and Bad Exorcism?

A key example of the interest in an "unspoiled" spirituality is represented by the current discussion about "shamanism." While shamanism originally described a certain form of spiritual experience in Siberia, it was influenced by the social structure of the societies in which it was created as well as by contacts with nearby populations, who transmitted cultural influences from China such as Buddhism (Shirokogoroff 1935), and the term is often currently used to denote "ecstatic," spiritual healing by any kind of traditional healer in any non-Western society worldwide. Moreover, the modern psychotherapeutic market offers a wide variety of ways to promote "trance" experiences via shamanistic rituals, which are being taught by members of industrialized societies. The "shamanistic" approach to nature bypasses the social revolutions and fundamental changes of industrialized societies and instead offers an "age-old" experience of nature, a nature that has not yet been subjected to capitalist exploitation. A common enemy of such movements is a so-called dualist rationality, which is not so much defined by its construction of hierarchies and its socially exterminating procedures as its critical reflection of "spiritual" experiences. With critical theory just located on the side of "dualist" rationality, however, the field is wide open for all kinds of religious experiences, including traditional ones. It is within this strange mixture of a "New Age" and a "neoliberal" discourse that one can experience a reemergence of Catholic exorcism and the religiously inspired healing of homosexuality.

However, there is truth in the proverb, "If two people do the same, it's not the same": while criticism of the "great evolutionary narratives" and the associated construction of colonial and social hierarchies as well as the exclusion and extermination of psychiatric patients are consistent with anti-colonial struggles, the revitalization of exorcism and therapies against homosexuality are clearly not. It was only in the last two decades that homosexuality disappeared from the major psychiatric textbooks as a disorder. Modern psychiatric theories, under pressure from critical gay and lesbian groups and professional organizations, revoked the idea that human sexuality can be classified as "normal" or "unhealthy." The strong stigma still associated with homosexual desires and behaviors in various parts of the world is implicated in the high rate of mental suffering that can be found among people oriented towards their own gender. Offering relief from such distress by trying to persuade homosexually oriented men and women to abandon their desires and interests and return to a "normal" kind of sexual interest in accordance with supposedly traditional Christian values merely reconstructs hierarchies that had previously been articulated and reified by degeneration theory and its exterminatory practice. There is a fundamental difference between a romantic and maybe naïve interest in shamanism, which (often arrogantly) denies and ignores cultural differences and social experiences of the populations who are exploited with respect to their spiritual traditions on the one hand, and a revitalization of traditional Western ways, which demonize and expulse "extraordinary experiences" (such as hallucinating voices or experiencing the insertion of thoughts from the outside) and oppress socially stigmatized sexual orientations on the other. While the romantic approach is at worst ignorant about the traditions it aims to exploit for the amusement of alienated Western populations, it still reflects some of the anti-colonial and anti-hierarchical discourses that had once shattered the dangerous invasion of "European rational superiority." This critical tradition is completely absent in current attempts to reevoke exorcism and exclude homosexuality; instead, it shortcuts a critical historical development and brings it back to its 19th century roots, including the moralization of behavior, the condemnation of social and sexual diversity and the subjection of individuals suffering from alienation caused by rigid concepts of "normality." Hence, it appears to be necessary to revitalize critical theories to cope with reactionary tendencies in current Western societies if the demonization and, ultimately, exclusion of subjects with extraordinary experiences or diverse sexual orientations are to be rejected.

**References**

Czihak, G. 1981 Biologie: Ein Lehrbuch. 3rd edition. Berlin: Springer.

Erikson, E. H. 1965 Childhood and Society. Harmondsworth: Penguin.

Evans-Pritchard, E. E. 1937 Witchcraft, Oracles and Magic among the Azande. Oxford: Oxford University Press.

Feyerabend, P. K. 1975 Against Method: Outline of an Anarchistic Theory of Knowledge. London: New Left Books.

Heinz, A. 1998 Colonial Perspectives in the Construction of the Psychotic Patient as Primitive Man. Critique of Anthropology 18:421–444.

Kuhn, T. S. 1962 The Structure of Scientific Revolutions. Chicago: University of Chicago Press.

Lévi-Strauss, C. 1962 La pensée sauvage. Paris: Librairie Plon.

McCulloch, J. 1995 Colonial Psychiatry and the African Mind. Cambridge: Cambridge University Press.

Mönter, N. 2007 Seelische Erkrankung, Religion und Sinndeutung. Bonn: Psychiatrie-Verlag.

Morel, B. A. 1857 Traité des dégénérescences physiques, intellectuelles et morales de l'espèce humaine et des causes, qui produisent ces variétés maladives. Paris: J. B. Baillière.

Olusoga, D., and C. Erichsen 2010 The Kaiser's Holocaust. London: Faber and Faber.

Reich, W. 1973 Charakteranalyse. Frankfurt: Fischer.

Shirokogoroff, S. M. 1935 Psychomental Complex of the Tungus. London: Kegan Paul.

# Chapter 3

# On the Notion of Social Pathology[1]

*Alain Ehrenberg*


**Introduction**

About 20 years ago, a French nurse said to a psychiatrist: "Doctor, help me to understand, people don't suffer anymore the way they used to!" For more than 20 years, French mental health professionals have underscored the increase of the "new ways of suffering" resulting from the transformations of the workplace, family, et cetera. They are new in the sense that they are characterized by the idea that people no longer manage to do things required of them; they display feelings of insufficiency regarding social ideals or constraints. People show anxieties of loss and insufficiency, and their anxieties are about self-image, narcissism and self-esteem.

In the conclusion of her book dedicated to depression in Japan, Junko Kitanaka (2012) writes that anthropologists and sociologists are now starting to go beyond the domination/resistance model. This model can be characterized as a sociological analysis, which is primarily political—domination/resistance being typical political vocabulary of power struggle relationships. But I must add: this is politics in a very narrow sense, politics conceived of by academics, a jeremiad denouncing social evils—the belabored self, emotional work and other falls of public man—without indicating concrete levers for action. Too many scholars have adopted what anthropologist Francis Zimmerman called the "mourning paradigm" 20 years ago (Zimmermann 1991:186). My perspective, which I have to admit is a minority report, is to propose an alternative to this hyper-political view: I approach the issues at stake in the mental health area more in terms of transformations of ideals or collective representations than of power relationships, that is, in terms of a Durkheimian rather than Foucauldian or Frankfurt School orientation. Collective repre-

---

[1] This chapter is based on Ehrenberg (2010a).

sentations are not constraints that come from outside, but are expectations that constitute us by affecting us in a *total manner* (Mauss 1968:308).[2]

Through psychiatric syndromes, many tensions of society are at the foreground. Most of the problems grouped under the heading "mental health"—depression, addictions, ADHD and others—tend to be subject to social and political concerns about what is right, fair, unfair, good, bad; they tend to be a soul-searching area of life in society and have become objects of intense and ongoing social controversy. The controversies at issue revolve around the argument that these conditions are in fact not only illnesses requiring treatment, but also social ills involving values and ideals inherent to our way of life. At stake are the values we attach to our social relations—in school, the family and the workplace, and by extension, in society as a whole.[3] Although these ills affect people individually, they also manifest a common ill or problem that is social, even sociopolitical in nature. This question of the value of social relations, of their human value, cannot be set aside: it is an intrinsic characteristic of these subjects; it belongs to their grammar. This is why one speaks of social pathology.

The idea underlying the adjunction of the adjective "social" to the substantive "pathology" is that mental pathologies are the product of our social relationships, that they reveal something about our mores and our lifestyles and that there is a moral, social and political lesson to be drawn from this type of pathology. At the end of the 19th century, neurasthenia inaugurated the tradition of social pathology: it was the first illness of modern life. Today, this topic is related to the widespread—and very confusing—idea in the social sciences and philosophy that there is a double process of psychologization resulting from a weakening of social links, and of a decline of public man in favor of private man. Partisans of this idea mainly claim that genuine society is what used to be. Sociology, in my opinion, has to go beyond this causal explanation. This notion raises the tricky issue of the relationships between changes in symptoms and personality, and changes in social norms and values.

---

2   Mauss points out that it is through the "physiological effect" that one identifies the social expectation.
3   For instance, for the UK see Wilkinson and Pickett (2009) on relationships between inequalities and mental health.

To try to clarify the notion, I will focus on the basis on which this widespread idea has been elaborated since the 1970s. This basis is made up of pathologies coming from British and American psychoanalysis: narcissistic and borderline pathologies, what psychiatry labels "narcissistic personality disorders." They belong to the category of "character neurosis." These neuroses are characterized by a disorganization of the personality and notably self-esteem problems, which didn't exist in "traditional" neurosis, the so-called transference neurosis—that is, hysteria, phobia and obsession—and by anxieties of loss rather than of conflict. In transference neurosis, it is both the superego and the conflict between what is allowed and what is forbidden which are at stake; in character neurosis, it is both the ideal ego and loss which are the problem. Today, psychoanalysts deem that most contemporary patients belong to the second category. They tend to think that they address less a therapy of the repressed, the one of transference neurosis, than one of the ideal, the one of character neurosis. In this shift from transference to character, depression has played a major role, but I want to address a parallel issue.

On the basis of this class of neurosis, two American sociologists, Richard Sennett in 1977 with *The Fall of Public Man* and Christopher Lasch in 1979 with *The Culture of Narcissism* successfully launched the idea that the individual has become narcissistic. This psychoanalytic notion has been successfully accepted as a sociological concept: a wide moral, social and political consensus has been shaped to claim that Narcissus has replaced Oedipus.

Sennett and Lasch raised a question on the basis of these pathologies: are we facing a transformation of individualism, which is turning against both society and the individual himself? I will approach this sociological transfiguration of the psychoanalytic notion of narcissism in the American context at two levels, sociological and epistemological.

At the sociological level, I consider it a narrative which shows tensions specific to American individualism. The issue is less the truth or mistake of this narrative than its success. It seems to me that its success in America lies in its anchoring into a style of rhetoric that the historian of American literature Sacvan Bercovitch called "the American jeremiad" in a book published with this title in 1978. The term is descriptive: it designates the political sermons by Puritan ministers of New England in the 17th century, which "joined lament and celebration in reaffirming America's mission" (Bercovitch 1978:9). The jeremiad is characterized as follows: reinstating ideal norms of the past, condemning the current state of the community, a prophetic view announcing that the gap between past and present will be filled in by a punishment sent by God, which is a correction. They made up an American ritual "designed to join social criticism to spiritual renewal, public to private identity" (Bercovitch 1978:11). On the other hand, at the epistemological level, as a tool for sociological analysis, I will criticize this narrative because it is an individualistic sociology, that is, a sociology which is trapped in the opposition between the individual and society, obsessed by a feeling of decline and of social dissolution and not a sociology of individualism, which goes beyond this opposition. To summarize my point: the fear of social dissolution is a common idea in our society, it is a social idea; the sociologist has to describe and analyze this fear as a feature of our society and has to go beyond it, as a sociology of individualism. This hypothesis will lead to the approach of mental health as a means of dealing with individualistic passions.

**Elements of American Individualism**

Its specificity lies in a category which symbolizes the American way: the self. Before being a philosophical or psychological concept, the self is a specifically American anthropological category, at least if one compares the US to France, where there is no such thing as a self, a category whose origins are social. It is a collective representation, a common idea in American society. Greatest social value is attached to this concept. It is an expression of a shared way of living which represents the automotivated individual, who is a fundamental common value of American society. It harks back to the Puritan origins of America, continues on to the Revolution of the end of the 18th century, and 19th century Romanticism, notably with its major figurehead, Ralph Waldo Emerson. While the American individual's first duty is to society (this duty was previously to God), the French individual's first duty is to society, through the state, which has obligations of protection toward the individual—the state being the expression of solidarity of society to any individual. Of course, the self is not considered alone, as an isolated entity, but is intertwined in a cluster of related concepts: self-reliance, which means trust in oneself and independence, and self-government, which designates the interdependent pairing of individual and community. It also refers to another pair of key values: achievement, which has its source in Puritanism, and equality, which results from the democratic nature of society and is conceived of in terms of opportunity. We French people value an equality conceived of in terms of protection. "Opportunity" is not highly valued, but is comparable to "protection" in the US: a secondary value. The US and France are like reversed mirror images.

The self, then, is not something inside the individual, but the interface between impersonal and personal (Bercovitch 1975); it is the common, what is shared between us. The self is the motor of this "restless activity" noticed by Tocqueville, and the crisis of the self is a permanent feature of American history. This goes back to the Puritan foundation in which the wrench of the self is a permanent ordeal faced with the double predestination: elected or doomed? To soothe this wrench, believers found in the "exemplar biographies" a scene for their dilemma and of their resolution. In *Auto-Machia* (1607), a popular piece of poetry of Puritan literature, George Goodwin wrote: "I sing my SELF; my *Civil Warrs* [sic] within" (Bercovitch 1975:13). This "narcissistic *liebestod*," as Bercovitch put it, is a swaying between fall and redemption. We will later again find this swaying in the tensions between "individualism" and "community," or between private and public happiness.

In the 18th century, this doctrine evolved thanks to Methodism, which added an affective and cheerful element to Puritanism: the authentic convert could take advantage of his life on earth, which gave rise to what Max Weber called "a culture of affectivity" (Weber 2003:241). In the 19th century, American Romantics used the tradition of the exemplary biographies in a new literary genre: the American autobiography. They celebrated their own self as representative of America. Ralph Waldo Emerson, the most famous of them, merged romantic naturalism with Puritan hermeneutics in an idea of the American self in which the personal and the common are intertwined. The relationship between the individual and America is as direct as the relationship between the believer and his or her God. I did not refer to the mortal narcissism of the Puritans by chance, because the picture Sennett and Lasch gave of the narcissistic individualism takes place in this Puritan tradition.

## The Encounter between Psychoanalysis and Sociology

The transformation of narcissism into a sociological concept results from the encounter between the main trend of American psychoanalysis, the Ego Psychology School and the exploration of the American character, the brand name of American social sciences since David Riesman's *Lonely Crowd* published in 1950. Two recurrent topics that have been used to criticize transformations of individualism until today first appeared in this seminal book: "personalization" and "privatization." This encounter appears in a social context that I will specify further.

In the US, contrary to France, psychoanalysis was introduced in the context of a global interest in psychology, a psychology which seeks to enhance the personal ability to connect with others successfully. For instance, Freud raised so much interest among American scholars that *The American Journal of Sociology* devoted a whole issue to his work in 1939, the year of his death. Another feature of American psychoanalysis and of the relationships between psychoanalysis and sociology in the US is the role played by the Frankfurt School, the Culture and Personality School and, more generally, culturalism. The issue of "personality" is a major topic of American social science. This was not the case in France, where the French sociological school considered the notion of "personality" and collective psychology suspiciously. In a speech given before the French Society of Psychology in 1924 Marcel Mauss asserted that collective psychology described the group spirit without the description of the group itself. He called it "the contentious discipline" (Mauss 1968:296).

The key moment unfolded between the 1930s, with the work of Eric Fromm and Karen Horney, and 1950, the year *The Lonely Crowd* was published. *The Lonely Crowd* is still the biggest commercial success of American sociology, and Riesman was the first social scientist to be on the cover of *Time* magazine after its paperback publication in 1953. His book was explicitly founded on a hypothesis formulated by Fromm. The Frankfurt School, the Culture and Personality School, et cetera, have contributed, among many others, to the American way of representing common life on the basis of the self-motivated individual. The concept of collective personality has opened a space of exchange between psychoanalysis and sociology, a space which is a sort of a division of labor: psychoanalysis being about individual psychology and sociology about collective psychology.

Following the publication of *The Lonely Crowd*, numerous studies on the American character and its changes were published. At the same time, several books by psychoanalysts popularized the idea that the character or the personality of the patient had changed. *Childhood and Society* by Erik Erikson (1950) or *The Quest for Identity* by Allen Wheelis (1958) described new patients who were no longer subjected to the same type of neurotic disorder as those of Freud's time. They suffered from identity disorders, from disorders of self-image, that is, pathologies in which social and moral ideals of the individual are core symptoms. Oftentimes, these patients did not show clear symptoms, but rather a vague and permanent malaise.

Here, I have to emphasize the social role played by character neurosis: this notion rendered psychoanalysis less strange, because everybody could recognize common social types through it. With this sort of neurosis, "psychoanalysts henceforth could not only speak of conflicts related to sexuality, but also of character psychology easily recognizable in daily life in striking descriptive terms. Organized around character and identity, psychoanalysis could enter in public space more easily" (Makari 2008:386).

The evolution of ideas on individual personality in psychoanalysis, and on collective personality in sociology, led to an epistemological and moral alliance between the two disciplines. The consequence is that both issues of changes in the normal and the pathological individual are elaborated interdependently. This shaped the "American jeremiad" narrative of the last third of the 20th century. The changes in psychopathology which appeared in borderline and narcissistic patients were the foundation on which a moral, social and political criticism has been built about certain trends in American society. Psychoanalysis has been used as a means of information on what is going on in individual reality. It runs deep into the self-conscious self, into this personality which is valued from the outside, but which is collapsed, psychologically speaking. It shows the disintegration of the self when the pursuit of private happiness and the pursuit of public happiness follow different or opposite paths, betraying the American ideals.

*Ehrenberg*

In 2000, an American political scientist from Harvard, Robert Putnam, gathered an abundant corpus of quantitative studies allowing the synthesis of trends in terms of strengths and weaknesses of social links. *Bowling Alone*, a worldwide success, empirically showed the following:

For the first two-thirds of the twentieth century a powerful tide bore Americans into ever deeper engagement in the life of their communities, but a few decades ago—silently, without warning—that tide reversed and we were overtaken by a treacherous rip current. Without at first noticing, we have been pulled apart from one another and from our communities over the last third of the century. [Putnam 2000:27]

During the 1960s and 1970s, American individualism entered into a crisis which expresses itself in a split between private and public happiness. This has given rise to abundant literature and huge media buzz on the following two topics: psychotherapy considered as a worldview and a new character of social life: the narcissistic individual.

This encounter between psychoanalysis and sociology happened in a context that I will characterize by two features: the first is what can be termed as the end of a liberal cycle, which started with Roosevelt and his development of public policies aimed to protect individuals and his struggle against inequalities; the second feature is the change in mores represented by the tide of sexual liberation, of valorization of self-ownership, the search for true self (authenticity) and by the movements of emancipation of minorities. These two features are intertwined because policies which aimed to protect the weaker categories of people contributed to the claim of the "personal." The American paradox is that a new individualism has developed thanks to state protection—as if America were like France—but this has led to a crisis of liberalism, which at the same time is a crisis of the core value of self-reliance.

Changes in mores were characterized by a new value first noticed by American sociologists at the beginning of the 1960s. Edward Shils formulated it as follows in 1962:

To a greater extent than in the past, the experience of the ordinary person, at least in youth, is admitted to consciousness and comes to form part of the core of the individual's outlook. There has come about a greater openness to experience, an efflorescence and intensification of sensibility . . . In a crude, often grotesque way, the mass society has seen the growth, over wide areas of society, of an appreciation of the value of the experience of personal relationships. [Shils 1962, cited in Turner 1976:1006]

The meaning and the value of what is defined by "personal" are not an issue of private happiness or unhappiness, but a public problem of justice and rights. Social movements of the 1960s related claims of justice and rights to the one of a recognition of personal value of the individual. "Personal," "recognition" and "experience": with these three notions rights are not only to be acknowledged, but also lifestyles—lifestyles aiming both to explore and develop the proper personality of every individual.

## Narcissus, or the Crisis of American Self-Reliance

It is in this context that the sociologist Philip Rieff published *The Triumph of the Therapeutic* in 1966 (Rieff 1987). By "triumph" he means that therapy is not only a tool to treat people, but a worldview which has transformed social man into a psychological man, this new personality which has signed the "failing of ascetic culture" and a "response to the absent God." "The therapeutic is the symbolic truth of the present age," and this truth is "the end of the vertical in authority" (Rieff 1987:xii, 40, 54). Psychological man, concerns about privatization, subjection to impulse and the loosening of community bonds: here are all the topics and concepts which will soon be the stereotypical concepts of the criticism of individualism in the US, in France and elsewhere. One is missing. According to Rieff, "The strange new lesson we have begun to learn in our times is how not to pay the high personal costs of social organization" (Rieff 1987:239).

On the contrary, Sennett and Lasch describe these "new personal costs" and they underpin their arguments with psychoanalysis. These costs consist of the idea that every individual self has become his or her main burden. Psychoanalysis has taught them that narcissism—and not simple egoism—is a tragedy, the tragedy of being locked up inside oneself, which makes the individual waver between a miserable and a grandiose self. Psychoanalysis allowed them to escape from moralism, in which Rieff remains trapped, because he does not perceive the tragedy of the individual. Narcissus performs the Puritan civil war of the self in which self-claim and self-denial are interwoven in a relentless fight. If narcissism is "a refusal of the self that centers everything on the self" according to Sennett (1979:270), it clearly stems from the dilemma of the Puritan who does not know if he or she is doomed or elected. The dilemma is reproduced in the oscillation between miserable and grandiose self, which is the hallmark of the lack of self-reliance.

The issue of affectivity is similar in Puritanism and in narcissism, according to Sennett: "The question: 'What do I feel?' becomes a genuine obsession." By the way, Rieff talked of "permissive" psychotherapy as "a permanent fixture of modern culture—a kind of secular Methodism for those who remain obstinately uncomfortable in their pleasures" (Rieff 1987:238–239). Narcissus is the secularized descendant of the man who lacks faith, who John Cotton portrayed in his *Christian Calling*: with Narcissus oscillating between the anxiety of emptiness and the joy of allmightiness, "It is the same act of unbelief that makes a man murmur in crosses which puffs him up in prosperity" (Cotton 1956:179). The narcissistic individual then symbolizes a crisis of the self, undermining both faith in America and faith in oneself.

Though these books are sociological, they are structured on the model of the symbolic analysis of the jeremiad: social criticism is connected with a call to moral renewal. Both are organized around strong oppositions: between past and present, between individualism of the past, "rugged individualism" and today's individualism, et cetera. In lieu of the divine correction heralded by Puritan sermons, it is a psychological correction which manifests itself in the painful narcissism of the self which is disembedded from community, a self which seems to rely on therapy only— 25 years later Proc was granted an analogous social status. These books are full of nostalgia for an American past which united the rugged individualism of the pioneers and the good neighborliness of the community (the French would not say good neighborliness, but solidarity). Their criticism is a ritual of celebration of America and its lost ideals of pursuit of both private and public ideals. They praise America by opposing the genuine individualism of the past to the current and artificial individualism of emotions, impulse, et cetera. Narcissism brings to light unexpected tensions coming from the emancipation of mores and a crisis of selfreliance that traditional individualism symbolized with its balanced alliance between competitive sturdiness, cooperation with others and personal independence.

Through therapy and narcissism, these authors gave both a form and a name to specific tensions of American individualism. Which ones? During the 1970s, the politics of progress, which developed under the supervision of the federal state from the 1930s to the 1960s, was called into question. As early as the end of the 1960s, this policy was strongly criticized, even by Democrats: it was wasteful and inefficient, increased bureaucracy and encouraged assistance, hence, dependence. "Affirmative action," designed to give advantages to minorities considered as groups and not as individuals, triggered strong opposition, because it called into question the moral individualism of personal responsibility.

In my opinion, the success of Narcissus is related to an association between a critique of federal intervention and the division of American society (culture wars, Vietnam war, etc.). Narcissus represented the end of a cycle of big government: becoming the operator of progress, the federal state, which gave up healthy competition, appeared as a nanny state for individuals. The crisis of liberalism is a crisis of self-reliance.

The strength and popularity of the arguments of Sennett and Lasch are due to the fact that they interweave two levels of analysis. First, they showed the crisis of self-reliance in strongly linking personal unhappiness to disturbed social relationships in a figure which is symbolic, because it unifies the individual and common evil in a very recognizable fashion for any American. Second, they blurred the traditional intellectual coordinates of the opposition between liberals and conservatives with a new synthesis which borrowed from the latter a moral critique of assistance and from the former the will to build a better society through social progress. They played on a variety of topics highly valued in American democracy and which represent America and its dilemmas: one clearly perceives the group rhetoric of the Americans, its main common representations. These narratives tell the fate of ability to seize opportunities when the covenant between the quest for personal prosperity and the building of the good society is broken. In this context, therapy is formulated as a stand-in for the lost community, and the community itself is perceived as therapeutic. Narcissistic and borderline personalities are variations of the difficulties of self-government, self-direction and on the shaking of self-reliance. Narcissus is the tragic icon of this crisis of self-reliance.

## Individualistic Anxiety: From Individualistic Sociology to Sociology of Individualism

The unhappiness of Narcissus is a narrative about the loss of the substance of life in common, which undermines both the individual and society. However, considering the narcissistic individual only is to focus purely on the dissolution of social links resulting from the loss of verticality; this leads to being trapped in the romanticism of the fall (*The Fall of Public Man*). The jeremiad is unable to progress past the democratic skepticism of social dissolution; it is powerless to escape from the idea of a loss of substance of the individual and society—that the world is disenchanted, that everyone tends to abandon the company of men, either by imposing oneself on it or in lamenting its disappearance. But there is a reason for this powerlessness: narratives which make up the American jeremiad are fostered by the skepticism to which they give form: they constitute a language game one can use to formulate the difficulty to make up society. The American jeremiad is part and parcel of what I referred to as the individualistic sociology at the beginning of this chapter. How can we go beyond this? And more, how can we do this without canceling the part of truth of this sort of narrative, truth which lies in the idea that this difficulty is a necessity in an individualistic society?

The problem with individualism is that we always need to go back to the basics, because one pronounces the word "individualism" as if it were something "individual," although individualism is a common spirit. Let us go back to the opposition of the individual and society. In 1898, Émile Durkheim wrote that one must stop confounding individualism with egotism: "Individualism . . . is not glorification of the ego, but of the individual in general. It is founded not on egotism, but on sympathy." He adds: "A verbal similarity could have given the impression that individualism necessarily resulted from individual feelings, then egotistical. But in fact, the religion of the individual is made up of the social institution" (Durkheim 1970:24). This means that behind the substantive, the noun "individualism," one is looking for the "individual" substance. Now this is exactly what, more than 30 years later, Ludwig Wittgenstein defined as "one of the great sources of philosophical bewilderment: a substantive makes us look for a thing that corresponds to it" (Wittgenstein 1965:1). Individualism means that every individual has equal value, because equality renders everyman similar to another—contrary to a caste society, for instance, where there is no such thing as sympathy for any individual.

However, one has to do justice to recognize the value of the belief and not reject it, because it tells us something true by highlighting the destructive aspect of individualism. Difficulty in making up society is part and parcel of individualistic society. What does this mean? In claiming a loss of substance of common life, the American jeremiad expresses a type of skepticism that one can term individualistic or democratic. There must be a place for such a language game, because it gives shape to individualistic anxiety; but, simultaneously, it must be struggled against constantly, because it prevents us from understanding how we make up society. Critics of American individualism continually repeat that one must struggle against individualism because it has become destructive—it weakens social links and creates new pathologies, like narcissism, depression and so on. However, Americans have always struggled against individualism. One of the main references of these critics is Tocqueville's *Democracy in America*, the first volume of which was published in France in 1835 and the second in 1840. What we learn from Tocqueville in this book is that Americans were already struggling against individualism at that time. He gave a framework to the issue of the difficulty of making up society; he gave it a locus from which it can be both recognized and struggled against. Let us follow his reasoning.

Individualism is created by equality, which gives the same value to any human being, regardless of social origin, which is why sympathy is a primary moral feeling in society. In one of his most famous chapters, he carefully distinguishes individualism from egoism: "Individualism is a recent expression which a new idea has contributed to giving birth to. Our fathers only knew egoism" (Tocqueville 1981:125). Why is individualism a creation of democracy?

Men who lived in aristocratic centuries . . . are closely bound together to something which is situated outside them . . . The general notion of fellow creature [of peer] is vague and . . . nobody thinks of dedicating oneself to the cause of humanity, but one often sacrifices himself for certain men. In democratic centuries, conversely, where the duties of the individual toward the human species are much clearer, dedication toward a man becomes rarer: the bond of human affection slackens and comes loose. [Tocqueville 1981:125–127]

And he adds that individualism constitutes "a natural . . . illness of the social body [that is, society] in democratic centuries" (Tocqueville 1981:132). By using the adjective "natural," Tocqueville means that there is nothing abnormal about this situation, on the contrary: "Feelings and ideas renew only by a reciprocal action of men on each other. I have shown that this action is quasi nil in democratic countries. So it must be created artificially" (Tocqueville 1981:140). The opposition between natural and artificial is a rhetorical way of saying that what we first see is the independent individual and then the interdependence of men. Consequently, in a democratic society, it is natural to remind individuals that they live in a web of interdependent social relationships, because they are independent beings from the vantage point of our supreme values. Because democracy renders the individual free in broking the great chain which closely binds human beings to something situated outside themselves; democracy has to struggle against individualism.

With his idea of natural illness, Tocqueville has opened a path in considering that the slackening of social links is a natural feature of democratic society and not an evil that destroys it inexorably. Why?

The answer is that we cannot have a democratic society, that is, a society where humans are presupposed to be free and equal, if links of dependency are not dissolved, for instance, between a slave and his master; but we also cannot have a society in general if people are separated from each other by the abyss of their freedom. This is the natural tension of individualistic and democratic society that Tocqueville has brought to light and that I call "individualistic anxiety." It is this tension that is formulated in the opposition between individual and society.

But to understand this truth comprehensively, we have to posit the issue of individualism in terms other than the opposition between the individual and society. The American jeremiad underlines the destructive dimension of individualism, which is a partial truth. It is blind to a central aspect of democracy that French anthropologist Louis Dumont has brought to light, enabling us to complete Tocqueville: hierarchy. For us, who are educated in the religion of liberty and equality, the concept of hierarchy is difficult to understand because it resembles inequality. Values of interdependence, which he calls holistic, are hierarchically subordinated to values of independence, the proper individualistic values. Interdependence does not disappear: it is embedded in independence. Embedded means it is part of it; it is neither independence nor interdependence, because interdependence is included in independence, but at a subordinated level. Without the holistic value, no society could exist. Thus, interdependence between human beings is as present as in "traditional" society. Dumont wrote: "Relationships between men must be subordinated so that the individual subject [or self] can be autonomous and 'equal'" (Dumont 1983:254). It is a necessity that individualism contains holism. This is why critiques of individualism are inherent to individualism: by reminding people that they depend on each other, they foreground the subordinated value of interdependence without affecting the supreme value of independence. That is what the American jeremiad does. It is a narrative which stages some dilemma of American individualism.

Now, considered not as a narrative but as a sociology, it is an individualistic sociology because it does not integrate the hierarchical dimension: it does not distinguish between the encompassing individualistic and encompassed holistic values.

## From Social Pathology to Passions

Narratives like the American jeremiad are a means of expressing tensions specific to a society. I would like to add another element related to the notion of mental health, which is at the center in this sort of narrative.

Philosopher Peter Winch, in *Understanding a Primitive Society*, explains that the magical rites of the Azande observed by the anthropologist Edward Evans-Pritchard "express an attitude to contingencies; one, that is, which involves recognition that one's life is subject to contingencies, rather than an attempt to control these." These rites "emphasize the importance of certain fundamental features of their life . . . We have a drama of resentment, evil-doing, revenge, expiation, in which there are ways of dealing (symbolically) with misfortunes and their disruptive effects on man's relations with his fellows, with ways in which life can go despite such disruption" (Winch 1964:321).

The centrality of emotional issues in our society can be described as a form of "mandatory expression" characterizing an attitude toward contingency or adversity in a global context where autonomy is our supreme value (Mauss 1969:269–278). Consequently, mental health is a major individualistic way of dealing with what the ancients called passions; it is the name individualistic society has given to passions. Mental health is about how we are affected by our actions and how we react to these afflictions, the social and moral equivalent of magical rites for the modern autonomous individual.

One should primarily consider the encompassing values and norms. In modern individualistic society, one of the most valued ideas is to become someone by oneself. Recently, this question of becoming oneself has changed. I would summarize the change as follows: we have witnessed a shift from the guilty and disciplined individual to the capable and autonomous individual. In the discipline-based system, the aim of behavior regulation was the docile individual, and values of autonomy, like choice or individual initiative, were subordinated; in the autonomy-based system, the aim of regulation is one's personal initiative. For instance, think of the shift from qualifications in the Taylorian/Fordian workplace to skills in the flexible workplace, and notably social skills with which an emotional dimension has emerged related to increased self-control. In both cases, the individual has to "self-control," to "self-regulate," but the style of social constraint is different. The meaning of discipline itself has changed: it is a means of training autonomous individuals capable of leading a fulfilling life. Self-discipline, that is, emotion and drive self-control, is a necessity in the autonomy-based system. Values and norms of self-motivation have subordinated those of mechanical obedience.

The history of depression incarnates this change. It accompanied the shift from guilt and discipline to capability and autonomy during the second half of the 20th century. It has progressively occupied the place of Freudian neurosis, that is, the pathology of guilt, and has become the shadow of the individual normed by autonomy. I will summarize the shift as follows. In a form of life organized by traditional discipline, the question was: am I allowed to do it? When reference to autonomy dominates the concept of society, when the idea that everyone can become someone by oneself becomes an ideal embedded in our mores, the question is: am I able to do it? Neurotic guilt has not disappeared; it has taken the form of depressive insufficiency. This shift of our configuration of norms and values has set the individual on an axis which goes from capability to incapability. As the cursor gets closer to incapacity, it makes one's inability to be good enough stand out (see Ehrenberg 2010b). In this shift, personal assertion—the capacity to assert oneself appropriately—becomes a core element of socialization at every level of social hierarchy.

We have been faced with new life trajectories and new ways of living, which affect the family, employment, education, relationships between generations, et cetera. Along with this we have witnessed the end of the welfare state of the 20th century. This change indicates we are living in a type of sociality where we all have to invest ourselves personally in numerous and heterogeneous social situations. Individual capacity to act as an autonomous self has become a major point of reference. It embodies our ideals of personal accomplishment.

This change modifies the relationships between the agent and his action: it increases the responsibility of the agent regarding his own action. The consequence is that everything which is about individual behavior, the mobilization of personal dispositions, notably the ability to change, in short, "personality," is a major social and political preoccupation.

In this sociality, individual subjectivity has become a major issue, a common question, because it emphasizes problems of self-structuring. Without this self-structuring, it is difficult to act by oneself in an appropriate manner. This was never a central concern in a society of mechanical discipline. The consequence of the shift from discipline to autonomy is a demand for an increased capacity of emotional self-control. At the same time, our social relationships are more and more formulated in a language of affect and emotions, distributed between the good of mental health and the bad of psychic suffering.

Self-motivation, self-control, self-discipline, self-regulation: there is of course a strong relationship between these notions and the place occupied by mental health issues in social life. Generalized attention to mental health and psychic suffering is a major reference point of individualization.

The main difference between traditional psychiatry and mental health can be expressed very simply: psychiatry is a local idiom specialized in the identification of particular problems. Mental health, because of its very large spectrum, is a global idiom enabling the formulation of the multiple tensions and conflicts of contemporary modern life and providing answers for acting on them. That is, mental health identifies problems generally linked to social interactions and attributes reasons and finds solutions to them. Today, mental health is not only about the struggle against mental illness; it is also a way of addressing multiple problems in ordinary sociality—in the family, work and workplace, couple, education, et cetera.

Mental health and psychic suffering are connected to the autonomy-based system as follows: change in our ways of acting in society, symbolized by the notion of autonomy, corresponds to change in our ways of being affected, symbolized by the notion of psychic suffering. Autonomy consists of an emphasis on the activity of the individual, but, at the same time, it is something to which one is subjected, which one has to put up with: affect, affection, passion, passivity, all of these words are about being subjected to or affected by something.

The value granted today to mental health, psychic suffering, affect and emotions is the result of a context through which injustice, failure, deviance, dissatisfaction and so on tend to be appraised according to their impact on individual subjectivity and the capacity to lead an autonomous life. In the mental health field, we find a genuine individualistic drama where mistakes, failures, misfortune and illness, all intertwined, are represented. Autonomy logically highlights an affective and emotional dimension, one which used to have a secondary value and occupied a subordinate place in a disciplined-based system. In this sense, mental health is a social form adopted to deal with passions when norms and value are entirely oriented toward individual action.

## Conclusion: From American to French Individualistic Anxiety

Narcissus has given form to a style of individualistic anxiety noticed by Tocqueville very early on. To end this chapter with a comparative perspective, I would say that this anxiety is formulated differently in the US and in France. Traditionally, we have no such thing as a self in France, if I may say. Rather, it is a secondary value. The equivalent social concept of self, the concept to which we give the same value, is the "institution." As Robert Bellah and his team pointed out in *The Good Society*, Americans have difficulties understanding the notion of institution. They write:

We Americans tend to think that all we need are energetic individuals and a few impersonal rules to guarantee fairness . . . It is hard for us to think of institutions as affording the necessary context within which we become individuals; of institutions as not restraining but enabling us. [Bellah et al. 1991:6][4]

We French understand very well what Bellah and his colleagues meant. In France, it is the state which incarnates the notion of institution. The best summary of French individualism was given by Durkheim in 1899:

The state . . . has been the liberator of the individual. It is the state which, when it became more and more powerful, freed the individual from his local and particular groups that aimed to absorb him—family, community, corporations, etc. In history, individualism has walked at the same pace than the state. [Durkheim 1975:163–172]

This sentence certainly sounds very strange to an American. In the US, narcissism appeared as a lack of responsibility of the self, a decline of individual autonomy; in France it appeared as a deinstitutionalization process, which meant a receding of the state, whose consequence, the exact opposite of American way, has been conceived of as an excess of responsibility on the self, an excess of autonomy. Here, the anxiety is the fear of an abandonment of society by the state, a fear that competition will then be unfettered.[5] This is another form of the individualistic anxiety.

**References**

Bellah, R. N., R. Madsen, W. M. Sulivan, A. Swindler, and S. M. Tipton
1985 Habits of the Heart: Individualism and Commitment in American Life. Berkeley: University of California Press.
———. 1991 The Good Society. New York: Random House.

---

4  This book was the sequel of Habits of the Heart: Individualism and Commitment in American Life (Bellah et al. 1985). This book clearly belongs to the tradition of the American jeremiad.
5  In La Société du Malaise, I compare the notion of autonomy in the US and in France because it unifies the American and divides French (cf. Ehrenberg 2010a).

Bercovitch, S. 1975 The Puritan Origins of the American Self. New Haven: Yale University Press.

———. 1978 The American Jeremiad. Madison: University of Wisconsin Press.

Cotton, J. 1956 Christian Calling. *In* The American Puritans: Their Prose and Poetry. P. Miller, ed. Pp. 171–181. New York: Doubleday Anchor Books.

Dumont, L. 1983 Essais sur l'individualisme: Une perspective anthropologique sur l'idéologie moderne. Paris: Éditions du Seuil.

Durkheim, É. 1970 L'individualisme et les intellectuels. *In* La science sociale et l'action. J.–C. Filloux, ed. Pp. 7–13. Paris: Presses Universitaires de France.

———. 1975 Une révision de l'idée socialiste. *In* Textes. V. Karady, ed. Pp. 163–172. Paris: Éditions de Minuit.

Ehrenberg, A. 2010a La société du malaise. Paris: Odile Jacob.

———. 2010b [1998] The Weariness of the Self: Diagnosing the History of Depression in the Contemporary Age. Montreal: McGill-Queen's University Press.

Erikson, E. H. 1950 Childhood and Society. New York: Norton.

Kitanaka, J. 2012 Depression in Japan: Psychiatric Cures for a Society in Distress. Princeton: Princeton University Press.

Lasch, C. 1979 The Culture of Narcissism: American Life in an Age of Diminishing Expectations. New York: Norton.

Makari, G. 2008 Revolution in Mind: The Creation of Psychoanalysis. New York: Harper.

Mauss, M. 1968 Rapports réels et pratiques de la psychologie et de la sociologie. *In* Sociologie et anthropologie. Pp. 281–310. Paris: Presses de France.

———. 1969 L'expression obligatoire des sentiments. *In* Marcel Mauss, Œuvres 2: Représentations collectives et diversité des civilisations. V. Karady, ed. Pp. 81–88. Paris: Éditions de Minuit.

Putnam, R. D. 2000 Bowling Alone: The Collapse and Revival of American Community. New York: Simon & Schuster.

Rieff, P. 1987 [1966] The Triumph of the Therapeutic: Uses of Faith after Freud. Chicago: University of Chicago Press.

Riesman, D. 1953 [1950] The Lonely Crowd: A Study of the Changing American Character. New York: Doubleday.

Sennett, R. 1977 The Fall of Public Man. Cambridge: Cambridge University Press.

———.1979 Les tyrannies de l'intimité. Paris: Éditions du Seuil.

Shils, E. 1962 The Theory of Mass Society. Diogenes 39(3):58–59.

Tocqueville, A. de 1981 De la démocratie en Amérique. Paris: Garnier-Flammarion.

Turner, R. H. 1976 The Real Self: From Institution to Impulse. American Journal of Sociology 81(5):989–1016.

Weber, M. 2003 L'éthique protestante et l'esprit du capitalisme: Suivi d'autres essais. Paris: Gallimard.

Wheelis, A. 1958 The Quest for Identity. New York: Norton.

Wilkinson, R. G., and K. Pickett 2009 The Spirit Level: Why More Equal Societies Almost Always Do Better. London: Allen Lane.

Winch, P. 1964 Understanding a Primitive Society. American Philosophical Quarterly 1(4):307–324.

Wittgenstein, L. 1965 [1958] Preliminary Studies for the Philosophical Investigations: Generally Known as the Blue and Brown Books. New York: Harper & Row.

Zimmermann, F. 1991 The Love-Lorn Consumptive: South Asian Ethnography and the Psychosomatic Paradigm. Anthropology of Medicine 9:185–195.

# Chapter 4

# The Religious Texture of Experience in Psychosis

*Ellen Corin and Ramachandran Padmavati*

**Introduction**

Research has documented a number of religious themes in the symptoms evidenced by people suffering from mental disease, particularly in the case of schizophrenia. More recently, attention has shifted to the protective role of religious beliefs and practices in coping with psychosis. However, because most of these studies are relatively superficial or limited in scope, we still poorly understand the way religious references are appropriated and used by persons dealing with the singularity of their experience of psychosis.

Anthropology has developed a richer approach to the very notion of experience, which is considered to be both subjective and framed by several levels of contexts: cultural, social, intersubjective and personal. And in the case of psychosis, this subjective context includes the general drift of the experience of oneself and the world associated with psychosis, the destabilization of the benchmarks of the world of common sense.

In their case study on spirit possession, Crapanzano and Garrison (1977) showed that religious symbols and idioms are appropriated in particular ways by individuals and that this process depends on the singularity of their personal and interpersonal life trajectory and their social positioning in the cultural scene. They argued that spirit possession idioms have a potential to articulate personal experience. Applying a similar perspective, we hypothesize that religious signifiers play a significant role in the lives of persons suffering from schizophrenia. This means that each narrative has to be considered from two parallel perspectives: one which focuses on the expressions and narratives involving the mention of religious referents and another which aims to resituate these religious references within the context of the broader life history of the person and the main challenges faced in relating to oneself and to the world. This radically displaces, at least at first glance, the need to decide whether the mention of religious items is "normal" or "pathological." The perspective resembles one developed by European phenomenological psychiatrists, who considered patients' words, reactions and behaviors as "phenomena," i.e., as the manifestation of a particular experience of oneself and the world, rather than as "symptoms" (Binswanger 1970).

## Insights and Questions Emerging from a Montreal Study

When researching persons diagnosed as schizophrenic in Montreal, we were struck by the recurring references to some form of religion, which was broadly defined in their description of their subjective world and called upon to face the frightening experience of psychosis. This was particularly the case for patients who had avoided rehospitalization for at least four years. In a time marked by the so-called revolving door in psychiatry—when many discharged patients are repeatedly rehospitalized—we wanted to explore the significance of "social integration" for the patients themselves and to identify what they believed helped them to remain in the "community." We explored systematically their social networks, their social roles and the social and spatial coordinates of their daily lives. In each of these domains, we were interested in perceptions and expectations as well as actual behaviors. We compared narratives of patients who were comparable at the start but differed regarding rehospitalization during the last four years.

In the analysis, some of the structural parameters of patients' reconstructed worlds were identified, as well as aspects of their meaningful texture. The social world of non-rehospitalized patients appeared to be characterized by fewer familial and social relations and social roles, as well as lower expectations in these domains and a relatively positive evaluation of their situation. This dominant "withdrawn" trend was compensated, to some extent, by elements manifesting an orientation "towards" the outward world, in areas differing from person to person. The expression "positive withdrawal" reflects the double orientation of the non-rehospitalized patients' subjective world, the relative weighting of each aspect and the positive connotations associated with withdrawal (Corin 1990). Their narratives reflected attempts to elaborate an intimate, protected inner space. Most narratives were colored by religious or spiritual connotations (Corin and Lauzon 1992), which seemed to help them find some peace or relief, as well as provide them some basic benchmarks for pursuing life.

Among non-rehospitalized patients, religious references tended to be borrowed from marginal groups and were often mixed with various esoteric or extraterrestrial signifiers; they evoked a kind of bricolage rather than an adhesion to institutional religious beliefs. In some cases, what was at stake was rather a global sense of a "presence" helping them to inhabit their inner world.

In another research conducted with recently diagnosed young psychotic patients (Gauthier et al. 2008), the importance of religious references in the descriptions of subjective worlds was also observed. Religion was mobilized in an attempt to express and frame the drift of their subjective world. Religious signifiers sometimes appeared to be absorbed within an array of psychotic symptoms; however, they also expressed a deep, intentional effort to tame, order and elaborate experiences. These expressive and restorative functions overlapped in many cases.

Thus, research done in Montreal suggests the protective value of religious references. It also evidences the solitary and marginal character of these attempts to construct a meaningful world at odds with the desacralized ethos prevalent in Western cities as well as in the psychiatric milieu. Would cultural sensibility to spirituality and religion reinforce—for the patients themselves and for relatives—attempts to deal with psychosis? To explore the interface between a drifting psychotic experience, the resort to religious references and the environment's influence in this context, we conducted parallel research in India, where religion and spirituality have a much broader presence in daily life. Multiple religions coexist in India, including Hinduism, Islam and Christianity, each one offering settings of cult, prayer and respite, as well as ritual healing: do people diagnosed as schizophrenic appropriate such a rich religious environment in their expressions and elaborations of subjective experience? And if this is the case, how far does a general religious ethos facilitate the communication between patients and relatives? In broader terms, does this resort to religious references help articulate positively an experience of psychosis? Do religious references contribute to the well-documented better prognosis of schizophrenia in India?

In this paper, religious references are considered in terms of their degree of flexibility within a religious frame, i.e., the possibilities of appropriation, and in terms of the window they open to an inner experience whose frightening character most often escapes words and communication.

**Context**

Research was conducted in collaboration with the Schizophrenia Research Foundation (SCARF), a WHO collaborating center for mental health research and training in Chennai, South India. SCARF activities combine the care and treatment of persons with serious mental illnesses, research, outreach programs and public awareness campaigns.

We developed a series of research projects with patients diagnosed as schizophrenic and their relatives. These studies were done either in the SCARF outpatient clinic or in Hindu temples and Muslim *dargahs*, places of devotion around the tomb of a Muslim Saint (Corin et al. 2004; Padmavati et al. 2005).

Broad, open-ended interviews were developed on the basis of a larger set of studies conducted in different milieus, including a remote area in Quebec (Corin et al. 1990), several ethnic groups in Mali (Corin et al. 1993) and in Brazil (Caroso et al. 1997). The objective of the first set of studies was to identify the "systems of signs, meaning and practices" locally developed in regard to mental health problems and to relate them to broader social and cultural dynamics. We explored the signs people used to describe the attitudes and behaviors of those who appeared to be suffering from some kind of emotional or mental health problem and for monitoring his or her positive or negative evolution. We also reconstructed their explanations and explored attendants' attitudes and reactions. Signs, meaning and practices were seen as fluid and moving realities and we tried to grasp their evolution through time, as perceived by the informants. We related these systems to social, historical and cultural contexts.

To explore the inner world of persons diagnosed as psychotic, we developed an open grid interview based on the same principles. The turning points interview approach systematically explores the subjective history of the problems perceived by patients and relatives (Corin et al. 2005; Gauthier et al. 2008). It considers the "turning points" of subjective histories by asking persons important details about patients' and relatives' attempts to cope with, explain and react to psychotic experiences. The open character of the interview allowed people to comment on what happened to them personally or to someone they were close to and to give extensive accounts of their experiences.

All interviews were conducted by one of the authors (RP) in the local language, Tamil. The audiotaped interviews were transcribed and translated verbatim into English by an independent translator. The accuracy of transcription and translation was cross-checked with the audiotape (by RP, fluent in English and the local language). These interviews were analyzed and compared in terms of signs, coping, explanations, reactions and help-seeking. They also allowed a more global qualitative analysis centered on particular topics.

To explore the roles of religion and spirituality in the expression and elaboration of the experience of psychosis, we focused on narratives collected in a pilot research study with young patients who had been diagnosed as schizophrenic in the last three to five years: nine men and ten women in their twenties coming mainly from a middle class background. While all women were Hindus, the religious composition of the male sample reflects the heterogeneity of the Indian scene: six were Hindus, one Muslim and two Christians.

## Results

In this paper, our main focus is on the patients' narratives; elements of relatives' accounts will also be mentioned when they concern reactions to patients' resort to religion. Examples are chosen to illustrate various ways of resorting to religion. Each case is introduced with the person describing his or her self-experience and experience of the world. These accounts help us to understand the individual significance of religious references and illustrate their degree of individual appropriation, as well as indicate the possible distortion of cultural elements for confronting the turmoil of a psychotic experience. The idea here is not that life circumstances "explain" a person's adoption of religion references, but that religious experience is embedded within a larger web that affects individual appropriations of religious signifiers. "Religion" was more influential in the men's narratives, which are the focus in this paper. Some excerpts from the interviews done with women are mentioned to reflect the similarities and differences of experiences.

## A Palette of Experiences: Men's Polychromic Religious World

All but one of the ten men's narratives include some mention of religious references. In some cases, they are struggling to resist a sense of deep subjective drift, but they still appear to be caught up in the tide. In others, resorting to religious signifiers seems to allow them to participate in a quest for a collective and reliable frame of reference, which minimizes the drift of their world. And in the remaining cases, the protective niche offered by religious places yields times and spaces of respite. In fact, these three lines of meaning interlace in various proportions in the life stories.

### Religious Signifiers as Enrolled in a Struggle

The enrollment of religion in a quest for personal significance is well illustrated in the cases of two persons.

The first case concerns a young man from a Christian background. Belonging to a very competitive extended family in which everybody has a successful, well-recognized profession and a good position in life, the young man is filled with a deep sense of inadequacy and great shame. He feels overwhelmed by an intense fear of the future, a fear of death and by a general confusion:

I'm not able to make it . . . it has become like an unproductive lifestyle.... I am afraid for the future, fear of death, of poverty, of being left alone. The mental thoughts are running . . . like a chain reaction—would it become this way, would it become like that. Would it be positive or negative, that kind of fear. . . . Future is black. Will I sit at home like a mad person?

In his case, religious referents appear in two different shapes. On one level of analysis, they color the prophetic visions that the young man describes as having appeared to him at three periods in his life: from an enigmatic promise associated with a mission to a degraded image that appears to mirror the drift of his world.

The first vision, which occurred when he was 17, expresses and responds to his questioning regarding the significance of his life and gives him a sense that he has a mysterious mission, a mission both appealing and frightening:

I was going to the church, I saw a man very beautiful, very powerful. He looked like Moses. Just when he was approaching he was filled fully with orange light and he was saying yes, yes, something like that: you are going to do it, you are going to do something. That time, some strong force attacked me.

In his comments, the young man sees the vision as associated with a sense of power and he interprets this vision as the sign of his exceptional destiny. He is fascinated by it, but something in him, in his very body, refuses the energy emanating from the vision. The image that appears to him clearly integrates biblical references, but the orange color of the light may also be seen as reminiscent of the monks and ascetics of Hinduism. In later visions, the enigmatic quality of the message is emphasized and words are replaced by a silence he tries to interpret. Its negative quality and invasiveness now take center stage:

He tried to communicate through his silence: you can do this, you can do that. I couldn't understand anything at that time. It was a sweet experience but after that, slowly, it started like a virus . . . now it has become very bad. A second time, this white light spread in my heart, then an orange light came in my head but both were rejected. The body shelves the light, never accepts light actually.

The visions and their messages continue to decay; the beautiful figure becomes an aged man and his promising silence becomes an incapacity to speak: "Everything started decreasing. So, the problem is—I don't have that light. . . . Now, I feel I have lost everything. Six months back he came again. He was very old and he said, 'Go, go,' something like that, but he was not able to talk."

On a second level of analysis, the same young Christian man calls to various forms of spirituality and religion in order to attempt to cope with his drifting experience. He repeats Vivekananda's *mantras* and starts reading religious books as well as books about psychology, body language and creative thinking. But this intellectual activity gets contaminated by confusion, which he believes exacerbates his troubles. At one point, he ran away and visited *ashrams* in search of moral benchmarks and a place of respite, but also in hopes of finding a place where his mission might be accomplished:

> I was interested in joining an *ashram* because I never had an idea of a good public life, because—no occupation and I thought of going to an *ashram* and concentrate on something. Spiritually I can do something good. I thought I am going to be something special, some saint or something like that. Something I'm going to give to the world. . . . I thought people will give me refuge actually.

He sees the *ashram* as a place in which he might be able to fulfill his exceptional destiny, where he could stand out. In response to his inner sense of chaos, the young man also searches for existential benchmarks, for meaning and for what he calls "moralization." This young man was asked by the Swami of the *ashram* to go back to his parents and to consult a doctor.

In this case, resorting to religious signifiers appears to have an expressive function and to be an attempt at restoring the experience: the use of religious signifiers may be seen as the young man's reaction to an overwhelming sense of inadequacy and as a reflection of his need for moral benchmarks in a subjectively drifting world.

His mother, a devout Christian at the Assembly of God, believed that the religious books only aggravated her son's problems. She does not acknowledge the religious dimension of her son's attempts to cope: "My son speaks a lot about religion but he is against religion." Her son's religious attitude is clearly at odds with her own.

The second example involves a young man from a Hindu background. His subjective experience is marked by the feeling that the general atmosphere has changed; he feels his life and his masculinity are being threatened and is overwhelmed by an intense fear: "On the shop, lot of workers were looking differently, wrong at me . . . like that fear came. . . . When that fear came, I went home, there was a doll, boy doll and I burnt it . . . a kind of fear came as if all males would die."

Overwhelmed by a feeling of helplessness, the young man searches for protection from Lord Ganesha[1] and looks at the god's image. One gets the impression that the icon functions as a point of reference, a potential

---

[1] Ganesha is a Hindu deity with an elephant head.

emotional container for his experiential turmoil. But this does not suffice to anchor his sense of self: "As soon as I burnt [the doll], I started looking at Lord Ganesha's photo. My time is not alright. My eyes have gone inside, my head is weak. Some customers say 'Okay, this fellow should die.'"

The young man becomes increasingly absorbed in the god's image. It becomes an obsession that invades his entire life. The family takes the young man to a priest in order to liberate him from this fixation, but the priest's rituals only produce a transfer to another object of devotion: "The priest tied a talisman and it reduced. After that again, I started to look at Meenakshi's [a goddess] photo."

Then, the vision fragments in disconnected parts, causing the young man to lose contact with the religious potential of the figure. This general process of decay now affects his very sense of self:

It increased, it increased. . . . Sometimes I would be looking at the nose, suddenly I look at the eyes—soon my confusion started. I felt as if I should look at it repeatedly, again and again. . . . I'll be looking at the fan, after seeing the fan, I'll look at the wall. . . . my brain would be, you are not in your correct shape, nose will be like this, my brain has become this way.

According to his mother, the deterioration of the web of protection that the young man was trying to establish was triggered by the deaths of a father's friend and later of his grandmother. When his father died a short time later, the situation worsened and his initial devotion to the gods turned into hatred:

Only after father's death it started again. It increased in the sense that I started disliking God. When my father was there, I stopped looking at the photo. After that, I started disliking God. I said God should die and I burnt all the photos. I started feeling very angry.

However, even in these desperate situations, he still associates a kind of protective aura to religious places, which he finds calming. When people say, "Okay, this fellow should die," he says he feels like going into the *pooja* room, a special secluded room for people to do their routine prayers.

In contrast to the previous example, the young man's mother presents her son as very religious and she encourages him to pray, to go to temples. She believes the calming atmosphere of the *pooja* room may be beneficial when he feels too distressed.

As in the first example, religious signifiers are engaged in a struggle: on the one hand, religious signifiers are employed to halt a sense of general failure and inadequacy, and, on the other, they are used to safeguard the self from fear and confusion. These efforts ultimately fail, and religious references appear to transform apace with the progressive deterioration of the person's emotional and mental states.

## Religious Signifiers as Moral Benchmarks in a Drifting World

A second series of examples illustrates the stabilizing potential of a more global reference to a religious ethos as a meaningful frame that may give significance to, and provide moral benchmarks in, a drifting world.

The first case considered here involves a young man belonging to a Muslim family. His narrative expresses an intense sense of fear and general difficulty in understanding the situation. He is overwhelmed by a sense of confusion and uncertainty: "I was frightened without my knowledge. . . only the fear was there. . . . I thought: What is the problem I have got? Why am I like this? I couldn't understand anything . . . only the confusion was there. . . . I felt that everybody was doing wrong to me."

In order to make sense of his intense experience, the young man constructs an elaborate system of interpretation related to the general significance of life, which integrates Muslim and possibly Hindu elements (for the importance of equilibrium). He interprets his present turmoil within a frame in which the bad time he is having at the present might be reversed later. However, his reasoning is marked by a general character of doubt:

Only recently I realized. It's to be well in life that I am suffering now. I have shown how bad a man can suffer. I have shown it to God. Loss here and loss there, gain here and loss there . . . in the other world. Loss here and gain there, gain here and gain there—so I should live well and show to the world and again in the other world also I should live well.

## Religious Texture of Experience

To reanchor himself in a shared world, the young man either surrenders to religious rules or performs daily gestures that give a routine to life: "What I did was according to Islam Laws—I read Quran, was fasting, brush my teeth with *Mishwa* Sticks."

Finally, the young man calls to a religious figure to legitimize his desire to withdraw from the pressures of the world and to protect an inner space inhabited by spiritual references:

There was a person called Noosa Nabi in those days, a prophet. . . . So I thought I should live a simple life. I thought I don't want to study, give the share [of] money I have to some poor people. . . . I wanted to stay in a hut and earn one day and spend for seven days with that . . . eat and the rest of time do worship, fasting and read Quran . . . do something related to religion, staying alone.

The resort to Islam in order to express and elaborate the experience is in accord with the young man's father's values. The father encourages his son to go to the mosque and to confide in a person doing rituals there. His mother also repeats that God is the only source of hope for him: "Only God can help him."

But despite this convergence, a significant gap remains: the young man refuses to go to the *dargah* with his parents, and the mother does not perceive the religious dimension of her son's behavior; rather, she considers his behavior as changed, bizarre.

In the other example, he perceives psychosis as having destroyed the benchmarks that organize human existence and give a basic order to life—that inform persons of what is right or wrong and help them feel at home in the world:

I used to think that everybody was looking at me. . . . I never knew what was exactly wrong or right. . . . I am not able to realize what my real talents are, my level of intelligence. . . . I am not able to judge, that is my major problem. . . . I was making my own rules: I shouldn't do this, I shouldn't do that. . . . I am not able to look out as a third person and say whether this is it, you are this, you have such capacity. All people have a basic knowledge, they have some amount of knowledge about all. . . . I think I don't have enough general knowledge to think about.

Under the advice of his mother, he calls to religion as a source of morality and guidance:

Mother told me to read *shlokas*, she was making me more devotional and was asking me to go to the temple daily . . . slowly I felt moralization was there. I was getting moralized. When I slowly went to the temple daily, I became more devotional and I started believing in God.

## Religious References for Protection

In another set of examples, religious references are mobilized in order to construct a kind of niche or space protected from the perceived violence of the outer or inner worlds.

The first case involves a young man from a Christian family. He describes an experience marked by great trouble and confusion caused by massive violence in childhood. His father would say about his son: "He talks too much for the little money he earns. . . . Why don't you die and all that, he used to say." His mother confirms that his father used to call him "a buffalo, eating without earning." The young man has internalized this accusation, which is expressed by a deep sense of guilt for not being able to take care of the family.

The violent family environment is reflected in the voices he hears. "I started acting as [a famous actor]. Even in TV, they would show some film like the way I was, exactly. . . . I felt to see things I thought in other people's eyes."

In a likely attempt to reconstruct boundaries for protection against violence and turmoil, the young man turns to the atmosphere of temples, in which people can be seen sitting or resting, sometimes for hours: "I used to sleep in temples only . . . in a place where there is peace and silence." He is aware of the reactions of others to this newly developed behavior but not disturbed by them: "People say, he doesn't like to go to the temples but now he sleeps there. What is wrong with him?"

The mother's narrative illustrates the polychromic character of the family's religious background, which interweaves Muslim, Hindu and Christian beliefs. The parents say that they only pray to Jesus Christ, but since God doesn't help them when they are in misery, the father remarks that there is no need to continue to pray to him and he prefers to go to the temple every week and do some *pooja*. They also recite *mantras*, religious formulas.

The young man appears particularly eclectic in his resort to religion. According to his mother, the young man went to the mosque and tied a talisman to counteract the approach of a demon. He also had a vision of a Hindu deity and his mother encouraged him to go to a temple. Although he likes to sleep in temples, he still refuses to accompany his parents and says that there is no need to pray.

A second example illustrates the idiosyncratic construction of a space of withdrawal as a means of protection against perceived or imagined violence in the world. In this case, the protected space is no longer religiously embedded. The young man feels that everybody is insulting him and that their sentences have a double entendre which escapes him. He therefore attempts to retreat into a radically withdrawn private space:

I'll sleep, cover myself and sleep. . . . I would sit with my head bent. I wasn't able to see anyone face to face. Then if they spit, I would have a kind of fear within myself. . . . I started feeling like staying alone. No hope seems to be left: I think that all is finished. Nothing can be done now. I am afraid of committing suicide.

In his narrative, religious references are more fragmented and partial. The narrative contains three brief religious mentions that do not appear to structure his lived experience in a signifying way. The first mention borrows from popular beliefs attributing mental illness to spirit possession or magic. When he consulted a faith healer, his face changed into a female face and the healer said that he was possessed by a woman. It seems that when he was young, a school boy did tease him, saying that he was like a girl. One may wonder whether this accusation remained alive in his subjective world and surfaced in this ritual space at a time of crisis. His second mention of religious signifiers might be part of an attempt to identify with an alienated experience of himself. He thinks that he might be one of Shiva's devotees,[2] as they were mad. The temple space is also mentioned but only as a convenient place for begging after his parents' death, as a

---

2   The Hindu god Shiva is part of the Trinity of Hinduism (Brahma, Vishnu, Shiva) and is known as the "Destroyer."

means of survival. In this reference, he borrows the imagery of the ascetics who use to ask for alms next to temples.

He describes his family as very religious, and his mother and sister used to go to the temple to pray for him. He comments that he objects to their actions, and accuses his mother of writing about him in her invocations at the temple.

These various examples illustrate the individual freedom of selecting and appropriating religions when attempting to confront and negotiate a threatening experience. Even if the religious references fail to resolve the person's life–world drift, at least in these first years of psychosis, they support an intense, elaborative process and indicate the degree to which these persons are engaged in an active healing effort.

There was only one narrative that did not contain any references to religious signifiers. It can only be stated that his mother was very violent to him, which is rare in an Indian context.

## The Experiences of Women

Dominating the women's narratives, at least when they are married, is their difficulties with in-laws, feeling unimportant in their role as wife or mother and the experience of moving back and forth between their in-laws' and parents' houses (i.e., they are sent home by their husband or in-laws and return to their husband's house when they appear better). Only three out of ten women mention religion in their story. They call upon religion for reasons similar to those invoked by men: to give expression to a subjective sense of drift, to attempt to heal and to find shelter.

The first case echoes the attempts of some men to express inner turmoil in religious terms. After a young woman's husband commits suicide, she becomes plagued by guilt and the sense that her world has turned upside-down. She reports a series of frightening visions and strange perceptions, like a strong breeze blowing in the room and whizzing sounds. She calls Rama's name and claims her innocence in regard to her husband's death: "All sorts of thoughts would come to my mind. I would tell my husband that I did not do anything wrong. I would weep in front of Rama's picture and cry that I have done nothing wrong. But the thought continued."

*Religious Texture of Experience*

She interprets another vision as indicating that her husband is in great trouble and she prays to God to help him. Feeling troubled by a great confusion, she asks the interviewer: "Do you get confused, Doctor?"

This woman's resort to religious signifiers in a time of great trouble is embedded into the general religious ethos of her family. Her mother says that they use to go to a nearby temple regularly and that she prays for her daughter. She sees her daughter's problems as a normal grieving reaction, keeping her integrated within a common world.

In the second example, religion appears to take a restoring or caring rather than an expressive function. This young married woman describes herself as extremely suspicious regarding her husband's fidelity. She also feels isolated from her family. She laments lacking concentration and her husband complains that she does not do any work at home and is aggressive.

She hears her mother's voice repeatedly telling her to come back home. Her only source of help appears to be religion and she does her best to integrate religion into her daily routine: she prays often, does *poojas* and reads *shlokas* and religious books. Her husband opposes these readings, but she comments: "If I do not pray to God, who else can help?" She wants go to the temple, but is afraid of losing her way: "When I go somewhere, something changes. I feel as if the road changes every time I go to the temple. So, I get lost." People around her perceive her religious activities negatively.

The third example echoes the longing for shelter found in religious places, which appears to be a dominant element in the men's cases, a shelter that the previous woman would also have liked to find. This third young woman lives in a very conflicting environment. She mentions frequent quarrels with her mother, her father, her aunt, et cetera, noting that going to the temple is the only thing that calms her and provides respite: "I would go and sit at the temple, near my house. I felt good there, not frightened."

## Discussion: The Construction of Experience

The research in India provided an opportunity to examine the role of religious signifiers within the psychotic experience of the individual. Patients' words illustrate their attempts to express an always elusive, enigmatic and frightening experience: to transform a "mere experience" into "an experience" that could be communicated to others. The importance of this distinction, rooted in Dilthey's writings, has been underlined by Victor Turner (1986) in his reflections about the anthropology of experience. He comments that experiences that severely disrupt routinized behaviors create "an anxious need to find meaning in what has disconcerted us, whether by pain or pleasure, and convert mere experience into an experience."

Experience does not develop within a void. It is shaped by individual subjective histories, relational and social contexts and culture at large. If the alteration associated with schizophrenia contributes to shaping inner experience, the experience also reflects outside influences, including relatives' attitudes and reactions and the availability of images, beliefs and symbols that may help express and articulate personal experience.

Cultural symbols and images are polysemic and their plural significance is open to a variety of possible appropriations. This is reflected in Crapanzano and Garrison's idea of spirit possession as an idiom having the power of articulating personal experience, i.e., inscribing it within a particular temporal, spatial, sensorial and linguistic frame and giving it meaning (Crapanzano and Garrison 1977). Case studies published in their book exemplify how individuals appropriate the polysemic elements of a spirit possession idiom and use them in order to face challenges associated with their specific life trajectories, social positionings or other aspects of their lives.

More globally, religious worlds participate in a dialectic that both objectifies and subjectifies (Lambek 2003). On the one hand, religion is embedded in elaborate systems of beliefs, symbols and rituals constructed by societies; it provides a common language related to issues of meaning and order. On the other, religion also concerns the most intimate texture of human experience in its confrontation with suffering, the finitude of existence and the enigma of life and death.

In our research in India, our starting point for considering the role of religious signifiers in the articulation of an experience of psychosis was the narratives collected from the patients. This led us to emphasize individual manipulations of symbols rather than purely describing a cultural system of meaning. The words used by the patients and the contexts in which they appealed to religion or spirituality emphasize the fluidity of religious references.

## Articulation of Experience through Religious Symbols

The Indian narratives illustrate the degree to which psychosis affects the basic coordinates of one's experience; they speak of the diversity of the religious signifiers mobilized in a time of crisis and of the individual character of their appropriation. Religious frontiers also manifest themselves as being fluid and crossable, particularly when one is searching for expression, help and relief.

At the level of expression, the terms used by most persons to describe the subjective experiences of the self and of the world indicate that these very experiences are perceived as highly enigmatic. It is striking to see the degree to which their words converge with Paul Racamier's (1990) comment that persons with schizophrenia are overwhelmed by deep disarray and experience the exhausting necessity, at each moment, of reinventing themselves and their relationship to the world. At that basic level, the words used by patients in Montreal and in Chennai are quite similar. We would argue that this is because culture imprints its marks on how we express, elaborate and confront an always elusive experience. But the extreme character of the psychotic experience might limit the potential for articulation offered by religious signifiers; there are cases, or moments, in which religious symbols and images seem to be absorbed by the drifting experience and lose their power to put a stop to the deterioration of the subjective world.

The examples also show that the expressive function of religious signifiers is closely associated with the need to inscribe one's life within a signifying frame that gives it direction and meaning, even if that meaning is essentially individual. Some persons speak of "moralization" when describing what they are searching for in turning to religion: they may seek the possibility of ordering their world or a source of distinctions and values that may redesign their existence, give it some stability and provide a source of a possible sense of self.

When one considers the issue of meaning, narratives indicate that the meaning in question concerns something larger than the experience of psychosis itself; it may concern the significance of the person's life and his or her suffering. Similarly, the "help-seeking" evoked in patients' narratives may not be limited to problem solving, but may concern the task of situating oneself within the world, as illustrated by a quest for "moralization."

Religious images or symbols mentioned by patients are situated at the interface between individual experience and culture. They might contribute to the articulation of personal experiences and their inscription in a shared cultural and social world. However, it is also clear that resorting to religious signifiers remains quite a solitary, idiosyncratic process; the meaning of images and symbols are altered and absorbed by the singularity of personal experience, which in some way disconnects them from their usual collective frame. Nevertheless, the variety of resorts to religious elements also testifies to intense efforts to counteract the turbulence. One can only be amazed by the ongoing efforts of persons diagnosed as schizophrenic to tame the inner turmoil and survive the deep destabilization of their lived world.

**Fluid Religious Worlds**

The internal face of the heterogeneity of the Indian religious scene is illustrated in the narratives from patients and their relatives; this heterogeneity facilitates individual appropriations of collective elements of the religions.

In their attempts to express and confront an experience marked by psychosis, persons move between different religious universes. Transcending religious boundaries was evident in the analysis of the help-seeking behaviors of relatives interviewed at Hindu temples and *dargahs* (Padmavati et al. 2005). This is in line with the fact that healing religious places in India generally attract devotees from various confessions and that this diversity is reflected in the vivid and polychromic atmosphere of these places.

In times of crisis, the search for religious signifiers resembles a quest that pushes people from place to place; the promise associated with the supernatural quality of the rituals and beliefs resists disillusion and remains open to a continuous transfer across religious frontiers. This confidence in the power of religious signifiers does not require adherence to a particular faith. In the case of psychosis, the necessity to call upon a variety of religions may also reflect the fact that the amount of personal and interpersonal disruption is always deeper than the "solution" offered by any single religious frame.

This fluidity may also be interpreted in the context of Lambek's remark that "the conception of religion as distinct, bounded entities closely follows Christian ideas that religions are mutually exclusive, that one has to commit to only one at a time." To this vision, he contrasts cultures where religions can be seen as a dimension of general ways of life rather than as distinct, closed entities. One can add that Hinduism itself is a very heterogeneous field (Dumont 1966; Madan 1987); the fluidity of gods' identities and characteristics, the often paradoxical character of their qualities (Doniger 1981), form a ground that may anchor that very internal pluralism.

Narratives collected in Montreal suggest one more hypothesis. There, the religious allusions of patients who had not been hospitalized for the past four years almost never echoed teachings of a particular church; rather, they borrowed from a large range of religious and esoteric frames. If they were attached to a religion, it was in an idiosyncratic way: they appropriated the particular religious images or symbols yet remained distanced from the community faith. One may suspect that this "long-distance relationship with religious signifiers" with religious signifiers creates a margin of space and a relative freedom which protects sufferers from being engulfed in religion. In Chennai, the protection of individual space might be an important challenge, a reaction to the paradoxically constraining caring and supportive family environment.

The Montreal research indicated the importance of protecting inner space for persons with psychosis, the need for a kind of psychic skin shielding them from inner and outer dangers. It suggested that various forms of withdrawal can be positive and that religious signifiers may support the creation of such a protected inner space and give it a significant texture. Narratives collected in Chennai illustrate that religion or spirituality may be mobilized outside of their semantic content, in a quest for withdrawal or in the search for a place associated with calm and peace.

Racamier (1990) argues that persons with schizophrenia cannot do without moments of retreat and regression, during which they withdraw into themselves, turning their backs to the world. One may hypothesize that resorting to religious signifiers can make the difference between a "negative withdrawal" within an idiosyncratic and private world and what has been called a "positive withdrawal" in the Montreal research. And in this regard, the Indian context offers richer possibilities than the North American one.

As a matter of fact, narratives also make clear that even if religion and spirituality retain an important place in India and continue to imprint daily life, patients' resort to religion often remains at odds with their relatives' religious behaviors and beliefs. It is seldom recognized as a positive endeavor, and patients often resist taking part in the religious efforts made by their relatives to help them. From the perspective of the relatives, the prayers and rituals they perform for the patient seem to establish a kind of protective net without requiring an active role. Relatives may mobilize a variety of religious references along their help-seeking pathway, which also strengthens their efforts in dealing with the situation (Corin et al. 2004). Even if patients and relatives are equally invested in the religious sphere, it often remains a site of conflict, as if patients need a certain amount of space between themselves and their family.

## With a Clinical Gaze

There are numerous reasons for being cautious in drawing conclusions from a comparison between data collected in India and in Montreal. The interviews in Chennai were done with a group of persons who were diagnosed as schizophrenic within a period of about five years at the time of recruitment to the study. The interviews were done in a clinical setting, the SCARF outpatient services, and were conducted by clinicians in a clinical setting; this context explains the ease with which patients disclosed the intimate texture of their experience. In Montreal, the interviews were conducted by the EC and by "lay interviewers"; they took place at the patient's domicile, in little cafés or in a clinical setting at the person's request; patients were met between two and five times. The duration of illness in this group of persons with schizophrenia was between five and fifteen years; and the data mentioned here concern patients who had not been hospitalized in over four years.

Thus, rather than comparing two homogeneous sets of data, we gained perspective from the characteristic differences in approach in order to deepen their significance in regard to psychotic experiences. If research had been conducted with longer-term patients who had more distance from the psychiatric services, the texture of the healing potential of religious idioms might have emerged more clearly or in richer ways.

As psychotic experience develops at a crest where individual and cultural signifiers intermingle, one may argue that clinical work should also be able to take into account these two dimensions or at least be attentive to their expressive or restorative potential. The psychoanalyst Pierre Fedida (2003) argues that the therapeutic environment should model itself primarily on the existential dimension of the lived trouble that affects the communication with the patient. For Fedida, the therapist allows the patient to appropriate his or her experiences, as the patient has to resort to words to express the subjective dimension of experience. And we know not only as anthropologists but also as psychiatrists and psychoanalysts that subjectivity includes the culture in which it takes shape.

**References**

Binswanger, L. 1970 Analyse existentielle et psychanalyse freudienne. Paris: Gallimard.

Caroso, C., N. Rodriguez, E. Corin, G. Bibeau, and N. Almeida-Filho 1997 When Healing is Prevention: Afro-Brazilian Religious Practices Related to Mental Disorders and Associated Stigma in Bahia, Brazil. Curare 12:195–214.

Corin, E. 1990 Facts and Meaning in Psychiatry: An Anthropological Approach to the Lifeworld of Schizophrenics. Culture, Medicine and Psychiatry 14(2):153–188.

Corin, E., G. Bibeau, J.-C. Martin, and R. Laplante 1990 Comprendre pour soigner autrement: Repères pour régionaliser les services de santé mentale. Montréal: Presses de l'Université de Montréal.

Corin, E., G. Bibeau, and E. Uchoa 1993 Éléments d'une sémiologie anthropologique des troubles psychiques chez les Bambara, Soninké et Bwa du Mali. Anthropologie et Sociétés 17(1-2):125–156.

Corin, E., and G. Lauzon 1992 Positive Withdrawal and the Quest for Meaning: The Reconstruction of the Experience among Schizophrenics. Psychiatry 55(3):266–278.

Corin, E., R. Thara, and R. Padmavati 2004 Living Through a Staggering World: The Play of Signifiers in Early Psychosis in South India. *In* Schizophrenia, Culture and Subjectivity: The Edge of Experience. J. H. Jenkins and R. J. Barrett, eds. Pp. 110–145. Cambridge: Cambridge University Press.

———. 2005 Shadows of Culture in Psychosis in South India: A Methodological Exploration and Illustration. International Review of Psychiatry 17(2):75–81.

Crapanzano, V., and V. Garrison, eds. 1977 Case Studies in Spirit Possession. New York: John Wiley & Sons.

Doniger, W. 1981 Siva: The Erotic Ascetic. Oxford: Oxford University Press.

Dumont, L. 1966 Homo Hierarchicus: Le système des castes et ses implications. Paris, Éditions Gallimard.

Fedida, P. 2003 Les bienfaits de la dépression: Éloge de la psychothérapie. Paris: Odile Jacob

Gauthier, A., E. Corin, and C. Rousseau 2008 Au-delà des modèles de pratique: Explorer la rencontre clinique en début de psychose. L'Évolution Psychiatrique 73:639–654.

Lambek, M. 2003 General Introduction. *In* A Reader in the Anthropology of Religion. M. Lambek, ed. Pp. 1–16. Oxford: Blackwell Publishing.

Madan, T. N. 1987 Non-Renunciation: Themes and Interpretation of Hindu Culture. Delhi: Oxford University Press.

Padmavati, R., R. Thara, and E. Corin 2005 A Qualitative Study of Religious Practices by Chronic Mentally Ill and their Caregivers in South India. International Journal of Social Psychiatry 51(2):139–149.

Racamier, P. 1990 Les schizophrènes. Paris: Petite Bibliothèque Payot.

Turner, V. W. 1986 Dewey, Dilthey, and Drama: An Essay in the Anthropology of Experience. *In* The Anthropology of Experience. V. W. Turner and E. M. Bruner, eds. Pp. 33–44. Urbana, IL: University of Illinois Press.

## Chapter 5

## Collaboration or Collision: The Involvement of Faith-Based Organizations in Mental Health and Suicide Prevention Programs

*Gerard Leavey*

### Introduction

Suicide is a major public health problem throughout the world. In Ireland it is the second biggest cause of premature death among young men. In recent years the suicide rate has dramatically increased, provoking local and national demands to reduce the toll. Various new approaches have been incorporated into suicide prevention strategies and key among these is the engagement of agencies such as schools and faith communities to monitor and refer people "at risk." The postvention activities of clergy should include pastoral work to assuage the suffering of bereaved individuals and to diminish the risk of imitative suicidal behavior among families and communities.

A considerable body of literature now exists on the need for collaboration between religion and psychiatry, suggesting that it is both logical and practical to co-opt faith-based organizations and their clergy onto public and mental health programs designed to increase levels of awareness, literacy and early intervention for people experiencing mental health problems and who may be at risk of suicide. However, the compatibility between these institutions and their worldviews may not be as easily reconciled. While clergy and psychiatry inhabit the same world of healing or, at least attenuating, human suffering, they also tend to view each other with a certain degree of suspicion and disdain (Bhugra 1997). That the latter institution has its origins in the former may not be enough to bridge the chasm between them.

The public health message that mental health is "everybody's business" is difficult to contradict, but in the case of the clergy it assumes that engaging with the secular world mental health and suicide prevention poses no threat to a theological stance. We undertook a qualitative study to examine the experiences of clergy in Northern Ireland and their attitudes to suicide. In this paper I argue that clergy are often traumatized by their contact with suicide, but more significantly, suicide not only exposes the loss of religious authority in contemporary Irish society but, apropos Davies, also leaves clergy lost for words against death.

Clergy are considered by statutory agencies as informed, vigilant people embedded in the community, advising and directing to services where appropriate.[1] However, the clergy have been viewed by some commentators as de facto frontline mental health professionals for many years, providing support and advice to people with a range of mental health problems, sometimes referring to statutory providers but often, not. Nevertheless, the value of the faith-based organizations to mental health promotion and early intervention should be obvious regardless of how effective they might be. Thus, despite the erosion of religious influence and welfare activity in the UK, the full spectrum of faith organizations continue to be well organized, contributing substantially to voluntary sector care provision and community cohesion; thus a significant element of what has come to be known as social capital has its origins in the religious sphere. It can be argued that this contribution has greatest impact in the lives of migrant and recently arrived communities in which it provides a substantial embedding and settling role (Leavey 2008). In the midst of rampant individualism and declining social cohesion and shrinking economies it is not hard to see why governments are once again more favorably disposed to partnerships with faith organizations (Birdwell and Littler 2012).

**Clergy, Mental Illness and Suicide**

At the individual level, many people continue to consult ministers of religion in preference to secular mental health professionals and this may be particularly so among minority ethnic communities (Cole et al. 1995; McCabe and Priebe 2004). The reasons for religious help-seeking behavior are varied, but these include personal trust and familiarity, a cultural-religious explanation of the problem (for example, spirit possession,

---

1 Not exactly novel, the idea of involving non-mental health professionals as adjunct carers has extended to hairdressers (Wiesenfeld and Weis 1979).

sinfulness and punishment) or fear of being stigmatized by contact with psychiatry (Mayers et al. 2007; Leavey et al. 2007). This contact means that if clergy were sufficiently knowledgeable about mental illness, they might recognize someone who is suicidal and be in a position to help them. Unfortunately, the few studies that have examined this issue indicate that clergy are given little or no training in dealing with mental illness or suicidal behavior, and lack confidence in referring to professionals (Domino 1990; Wang, Berglund and Kessler 2003; Weaver 1995). Importantly also, clergy have an important role in dealing with problems that may arise in the aftermath of suicide or a suicide attempt.

In many communities, clergy have influence on public opinion, leading, and in some cases challenging, attitudes and beliefs. Here, the long-standing but now diminished religious perspective on suicide has particular significance. Religious abhorrence in the Christian tradition dates back to St. Augustine and St. Aquinas. Thus, the Old and New Testaments make few references to suicide and these tended to be matter-of-fact reporting, devoid of any moral significance. From the second millennium onwards the Christian Church's attitude to people who take their own lives is distinguished by vehement detestation of the act and also of the actor who is deemed to have sinned against family, community and God. Life as a gift from God is his alone to dispose of; thus, suicide was regarded as a rejection of God's grace. Moreover, suicide was a sin which always precluded absolution—to kill oneself was a death without receiving confession, meaning that it could never be forgiven. For several centuries, the consequence for the suicide and his or her family was disastrous and profound. The suicide was denied a burial in consecrated ground, and often interred at the crossroads. The suicide's family were often stigmatized, ostracized and severely punished collectively with a loss of economic and civil rights. Similarly abhorred in the Muslim and Jewish traditions, the soul of the suicide was believed to wander for eternity. While a more compassionate view of suicide emerges in the 19th century through an increasing appreciation of the role of mental illness as a factor in suicidal behavior, a religiously informed anxiety about, and distaste of, suicide appear to remain entrenched in many sectors of society. Therefore, again it would seem appropriate that clergy are involved in some way in the softening of such attitudes and shaping or conditioning a more sympathetic environment for bereaved family members. Thus, postvention strategies may be targeted at people who have been affected by suicidal behavior and bereaved friends or family members, vulnerable to mental disorder and the development of suicidal tendencies.

It seems likely that for the reasons which I have outlined above, several national and regional suicide prevention and postvention strategies have indicated a role for faith-based organizations and their clergy. However, like many advocates for FBO involvement in mental health care generally, the complexity of clergy involvement is seldom acknowledged (Leavey and King 2007). The advocates for religious involvement fail to state the extent to which FBOs want to be involved in health and suicide prevention activities, what these activities might entail, what resources might be needed and what sort of difficulties this involvement might create for clergy and faith-based organizations? Such strategies assume a universal theological stance on mental illness and suicide and, further, appear blind to the risks and dangers that the envisaged collaborations hold for both sides in the partnership (Leavey and King 2007). In Northern Ireland a considerable level of government funding has been pumped into public health initiatives in an attempt to lower the suicide rates. The strategy also outlined the need for FBO involvement but gave no indication what this would entail. In 2008 and 2009 we undertook a study to examine clergy needs in dealing with suicide in their communities and congregations (Leavey, Rondon and McBride 2011).

In this paper I wish to elaborate on the findings presented in a previously published paper by specifically locating the dangers and risks for clergy consequent of faith organizations' compromise with secularism in the context of suicide. Presenting this study at the "International Conference on Religion, Healing and Psychiatry" (in Münster 2012) I suggested that the dominant pastoral response of clergy to suicide may be one of silence. At the pastoral level, compassion for the individual and those bereaved by suicide has replaced the traditional public theological condemnation of suicide but has left many clergy with discomfiture about the declawing of religion. I argue that secularism is both cause and effect of the loss of religious authority. Thus, the swing toward a secular psychological explanation of suicide lessens or censors religious opprobrium toward the actor and it also diminishes the authority of the religious voice when it perhaps might be expected to be at its loudest.

## The Study

We recruited people from a range of denominations to take part in the in-depth interviews. These were conducted with 39 ministers from the Catholic Church, Church of Ireland (Anglican Communion), Presbyterian Church in Ireland, Free Presbyterian and Methodist Church. Although we also interviewed Hindu, Jewish and Muslim representatives, these are not discussed here. The interviews were conducted with the use of a topic guide, which covered areas such as the participants' views on, and experiences of, mental illness and suicide in the community, their explanatory models of suicide, dealing with families bereaved by suicide and the barriers to pastoral care. The audiotaped interviews were transcribed verbatim and analyzed using a software package for qualitative data (Atlas-ti). For a full account of the study and analysis see (Leavey et al. 2008).

## The Impact of Suicide on Clergy

All of the participants in the current study had been involved in the pastoral care of families following suicide and several have had to deal with multiple suicides within their communities. In the close-knit rural and semi-rural areas of Northern Ireland, the suicide victims and their families were well-known to the clergy, sometimes neighbors. In a number of cases, clergy had been in contact with distressed people, sometimes providing long-term pastoral care, who then go on to take their own lives. In other cases, clergy were called upon to visit the suicide scene.

> I found that terribly torturesome and traumatic because he had nobody—nobody to say goodbye to him and nobody to console him. But it would also have affected me from the point of view of the violence of it because it was just a really angry statement at that place.

In the following quote a Catholic priest recalls his visit to the sight of a young man hanging from a tree in a secluded park, the small but significant details of which shatter his own assumptions about the act as a cry for help; that is, a belief he tenuously nurtured that ultimately no one ever really intends to kill themselves.

> I said the prayers and I anointed him and when I went to anoint his hands . . . and his two hands were closed tight in the jeans pockets. And I remember at that

moment realizing he meant to do this. You know he didn't want to save himself. It was that realization that it was so definite, final, purposeful . . . And I remember being so taken aback by that—that he really meant to do this. You'd often hear it was a cry for help. And I have to say that changed my whole outlook on a cry for help. At that moment it really changed my whole thought on that term.

However, it is not just the direct impact of witnessing death by suicide that produces stress for clergy, but also the complications of ministering to families in a pluralist society, which has not a unified religious belief, even within the same family, and no singular response that can accommodate the spiritual needs of all those impacted. Some family members do not believe in or perhaps feel abandoned by God. Importantly, clergy note the destabilization of families in contemporary society—fractured and made fragile by a range of problems, which then are often made visible following the suicide; schisms erupt into accusations about motivations and causes of suicide. From the clergy interviews, such scenarios are commonplace and leave the clergy feeling bewildered and disturbed as they try to negotiate their way through family anger and guilt. Underlying some suicides are difficult, unpleasant behaviors and/or in other cases, problematic life histories of alcohol and drug misuse arising from sexual abuse and family dysfunction. Clergy sometimes are aware of these "background factors"; in other cases they are not, but in all cases clergy inevitably become quickly aware of family secrets and splits. Often too, family members attempt to pull clergy into partisanship. Getting the balance right in terms of what can be said to families without upsetting somebody is a major problem. Importantly, while the pastoral role is complicated by the heightened sensitivities thrown up by suicide, clergy in general are seldom provided with specific training in mental illness or suicide.

Of course, dealing with suicide, and families bereaved by suicide, is distressing for most professionals even where training and support is provided, but clergy are expected to understand and deal with this most complex of situations purely from a religious framework, which as we have suggested is often no longer tenable. This leaves them further distressed by a sense of incompetence and inadequacy, exacerbated by the fiction that a solid personal religious strength alone will help clergy to work through life's problems and suffering. To succumb to burnout and depression is, perhaps, an indication to oneself and perhaps others that one's faith is

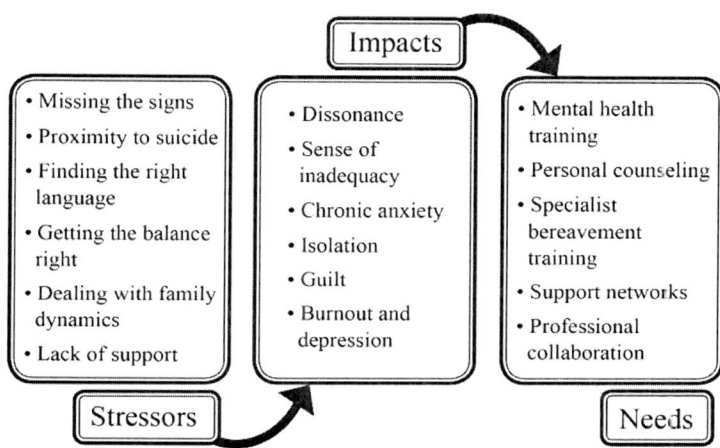

*Figure 1: Stressors, impacts and needs of clergy in dealing with suicide.*

insufficiently robust. Clergy, particularly Catholic priests, described their own isolation and loneliness and hinted at the widespread prevalence of distress among their colleagues. Others, such as this Presbyterian minister, described their own "dark nights of the soul":

During that time when I was depressed I went through a time, a particular evening actually, when I suppose the only way that you could describe it was that fear of death was gone and there was a kind of blackness descended over me and if I hadn't lifted the phone to speak to someone I mightn't be here today.

Figure 1 (above) provides an overview of the main stressors, impacts and needs of clergy in the context of suicide in their communities.

### Clergy Causal Attributions for Suicide

The causal attributions for suicide given by the clergy are similar to those commonly suggested by members of the general population. That is, these are explanations that tend to cover the personal and the social, the universal and the local—the latter encompassing the end of the Northern

Ireland conflict in which the external threat of violence and death that once demanded and underpinned community cohesion is now removed. What is interestingly different perhaps is that the clergy tended to offer explanations that are not that dissimilar from those of the sociologists, and while sociologists might not adopt a value position on individualism, materialism and secularism, they might concur that these phenomena fuel the rise in suicide rates. Ignoring psychological explanations, Durkheim asserted that suicide is primarily sociological in that societies with high levels of solidarity and integration produce less suicidal behavior than individualistic societies (Stack 2000). Where faith groups might differ from Durkheim is his assertion that the religious association with suicide deterrence had little to with doctrinal injunction but rather was a by-product of collective strength found in religious communities (Durkheim 1897).

Most commonly, whatever the background social or personal factors precipitating the suicide act, clergy suggested that, ultimately, suicide is the consequence of mental illness and, therefore, the act should not be seen as a voluntary commission. Moreover, only the omniscient God can fully know if the person suffered from mental illness and his or her fellow human beings are not in a position to judge. While suggesting that there are a number of more "hardline" evangelical churches which continue to hold absolutist views on suicide, most Christian traditions no longer adopt a punitive stance—denying burial rites and the like.

However, while clergy argue that a more compassionate response to suicide is now universally accepted within mainstream churches, ensuring that families are cared for rather than alienated by the church, there is also disquiet among them that perhaps the theological views have drifted in the direction of suicide acceptance. Thus, the contemporary churches' compassion in suicide is not without its ambivalence. Many clergy will argue that the churches have allowed prevalent liberal societal attitudes to determine the church response. As this Presbyterian minister argues, a harsher theological line on suicide may be more of a deterrent:

I have to say, first of all, that suicide is a sin . . . "Thou shalt not kill" . . . And if that was more fully recognized that it was wrong then there might be fewer suicides. I know that suicide is no longer a crime. We are living in a secular society where people are saying to themselves, "well, if it's not a crime, then it's all right." . . . Are we saying to people that if you do this, then we will have nothing but pity for you? Are we encouraging people to caress their own self-pity?

This kind of critical questioning of suicide tolerance is expressed by various clergy but always cautiously. At the very least, there is widespread clergy ambivalence on suicide. As we have suggested, the clergy should have an important role in suicide prevention and postvention activities, particularly so in shaping moods and attitudes in religious communities. And, even where religious attendance adherence is in decline, as in Ireland, the rituals of church are still sought by community members to channel and articulate grief. While tragedies, commonly sudden violent or accidental deaths, create an optimum vantage point for collective mourning and religious solace, suicide response is conflictual, the compassion guarded and muted. A leitmotif running through these interviews was that of "sitting in silence"—"just being there with the family"—which may be interpreted as an appropriate response to the vacuum created by suicide. But given the clergy anxiety about liberalizing theology, we may also consider it as a general silencing of the churches as they struggle to find a meaningful response to what is regarded by many as a suicide epidemic in many communities and is testament to a recognition of failure—personal, social, political and spiritual—that permeates the collective consciousness of suicide, and where the disposition of many clergy is toward outright condemnation, they find only a weakening of authority to assert abhorrence. It is often difficult to tap into the official line of faith organizations with regard to suicide—partly because there often is none. While clergy may fall back upon an exculpatory explanation of individual madness, that is, the person took their own life because they lacked personal agency though illness, they also suggest that this happens in the context of a societal madness, and once again I suggest that they have an affinity with sociologists—there is the anomie created by individualism, consumerism and secularism and therefore shaping the environment in which suicide becomes more possible. Crucially, although clergy recognize that they have an unavoidable role in dealing with depressed and suicidal people, they also have a distinct sensitivity regarding the sanctity of life, a disposition or worldview, which makes them lean more toward Augustine than Freud. The disposition of many clergy within mainstream churches toward suicide is a theological abhorrence that may be relatively unchanged since Aquinas. Importantly, the disjunction between what is expected of clergy and what they can fulfill develops into an overwhelming sense of guilt and failure (Louden and Francis 2003). The lack of support structures within the churches leads to further vocational attrition. Today, increasing numbers of clergy experience burnout and stress—it is a subject that they tend not to discuss between themselves and it is not something that the church authorities have done very much about (Weaver et al. 2002). There remains within the religious institutions a form of stoicism about the ability to endure suffering—and a correlational belief that it betrays a sign of spiritual weakness to experience depression.

## Discussion

The nature of secularism and the extent of its spread continue to be debated in sociology. If defined as a loss of a religious influence in the public sphere and cultural activity, then secularism would appear to be a reality in much of Europe. If, however, defined in terms of spiritual beliefs, the transcendent or supernatural, then the case for secularism is on less secure ground (Stark and Bainbridge 2002). However, more relevant to the argument presented here, secularism has impinged on theology and church activity in several interlocking fields. In this I restrict myself to Christianity rather than faith groups generally. The first factor relates to the relationship between church and state agencies in the provision of services, the demands of professionalism in pastoral care and the impact of such change on religious identity of clergy. The second field relates to the loss of the religious voice, which in liberal mainstream churches appears to have been surrendered in contemporary society, a trade-off that allows pastoral compassion to the individual but at the expense of public religious authority.

## Religion and Welfare

Although healing, education and welfare have been central activities of organized religion for millennia, they virtually disappeared from church life by the end of the 20th century. Thus, among European countries Prochaska (2006) perceives an inverse correlation between high levels of state welfare activity and low levels of religious adherence. In this vein he argues that the Church of England significantly contributed to their decline as an active presence in British life and in civic consciousness through their own embrace of government intervention as the only realistic means of addressing social ills. The Church, in doing so, unwittingly endorsed a "collectivist secular world without a redemptive purpose," which replaced a patchy, often amateurish, provision of welfare and education based on voluntary effort with a strategic, centrally coordinated effort that was universal and professional—at least, in design if not entirely in outcome.

An unintended consequence of this shift has been the significant erosion of social capital nurtured by the Church, an active commitment to help one's neighbors and community. However, state–church relationship in the late 20th century has shifted; encouraged by a diminishing economic base and an increasingly dependent elderly population, Western economies face a reduction in state control of welfare and are more amenable to a plural economy of provision in this and other sectors. This opens the door to a return of faith-based activism in areas usually the domain of government. Where there is consonance between the secular government message and that of the religious institutions, the relationship seems relatively straightforward; social cohesion, nonviolence and inter-faith dialogue are recurrently popular and commonly accepted themes. More contentious for some faith organizations are the restraints posed by equality legislation on matters related to sexuality and abortion, for example, or assisted suicide. A degree of ostensible neutrality on the part of the churches is needed if they are to maintain their voluntary sector activities. But, this kind of neutrality may be dissonant with deep or core organizational values and likely to damage relationships between the organization and their congregations and ministers. The second strand of this argument lies with the problems created by the uneasy fit between secular professionalism and what we might describe as the spiritual habitus of ministers to manage human suffering that may not be compatible with psychological precepts.

**Religion and Psychiatry**

The management of mental health problems among congregation members may leave clergy in an invidious position in that they struggle to find relevance in modern pastoral ministry knowing that if they drift beyond the spiritual boundary into the territory of psychological engagement, they rapidly become mired in their own acknowledged incompetence. There is a crisis in ministry and it is not simply the decline in church going; in almost all interviews with clergy they admit that they are completely unprepared for the problems now confronting them on a regular basis: the domestic violence, community and family breakdown, sexual abuse, alcoholism and drug use. They struggle to have relevance in the midst of the contemporary human condition and feel that what their communities expect from them is much more than spiritual advice or consolation. This tends to require a much greater degree of psychological knowledge and skill than they possess—and a much lower emphasis on the spiritual or other worldly dimensions. Clergy often struggle to get the balance right: "I can't be a social worker in a dog collar," said one priest I interviewed in London, as he emphasized the concern about drifting outside his spiritual competencies (Leavey, Loewenthal, and King 2007). Research by Mason et al. (2011) in America which examined clergy attitudes to pastoral care in suicide found similar concerns about maintaining boundaries between secular psychology and religious care. Among clergy there remains an anxiety about the different beliefs and values held by psychiatry and a still pervasive view that religion is pathologized by its practitioners. Of course, an anxiety about a perceived hegemony of the psychiatric institution in all areas of human wrongdoing and suffering extends beyond the religious field; other voices articulate fears that matters of conduct and morality are too easily annexed by medicine as matters of pathology and treatment.

This anxiety persists. Charles Taylor in his book *A Secular Age* (2008) argues that a feature of modern culture and its sense of human innocence is the transfer of so many issues which used to be considered moral into a therapeutic register. What was formerly sin is often now seen as sickness. This is the triumph of the therapeutic as Taylor terms it and which he suggests has a paradoxical effect—for although "it seems to involve an enhancement of human dignity [it] can actually end up abasing it." The shift in the hermeneutic from the spiritual to the therapeutic, he suggests, removes the heroic narrative of struggle over our innate sinfulness but only replaces it with a pathology that is manipulated and treated by others. It is not that Taylor longs to bring us back to a belief in sin and evil, but that as a "total metaphysic" it risks generating perverse results—further stifling the spirit within us or "fixing other incapacities more firmly on us" (2008:623). His point here is not that distant from the views of the clergy on suicide.

## No Words against Death

Functionalist theories from Durkheim onwards provide an understanding of how death rituals facilitate community healing and reintegration. Moreover, the transcendence of death is central to many of the world religions, with life after death surely promising the greatest of all compensators. However, Bloch (Bloch and Parry 1982; Bloch 1992) argued that death rituals are much more than simply supporting the reconstitution and reintegration of society following death; instead death rituals act as catalysts, empowering and energizing the survivors to push forward. In *Death, Ritual and Belief*, Douglas Davies (2002) suggests that by extension, death rites create an energy that benefits society and adds to human self-awareness and the building of identity. Thus ritual performances challenge the potential oblivion of death and, consequently, the meaningless of life, reestablishing and/or reconstructing the identity of the deceased within wider social and meaningful frameworks and thus permit continuity for those left behind. Words against death, as he suggests, are performative utterances against death, the use of rhetoric as persuasive speech to reassure the bereaved that they will be comforted, be healed, to "move on," in colloquial terms or that death may have been a release from suffering, for example. Words against death as Douglas argues are essential to Christian theology and ritual. Thus, baptism and the Easter rituals, for example, only have meaning in the acceptance that death has been conquered and that this continues to be restated. However, such a recognition of conquest requires a level of mutual agreement that is now unreliable. The lack of shared meaning on death and religion means that the clergy are no longer with confidence able to provide a singular explanation that covers all emotional and cognitive needs. Thus, while suicide ruptures assumptive worlds, in doing so it also provokes guilt, shame and recrimination in intensified form and expression, which projects the response of the bereaved and the community beyond what is experienced in "normal" death. The theological stance of the past meant that the event of suicide in the community was quietly and quickly concealed, its memory left unspoken. In contemporary Ireland and elsewhere the shattering consequences of suicide have become the source of political anxiety and public health intervention. And, regardless of the utility, there are very few hushed voices in this matter. The community, disquieted and demanding action, also finds the church and the clergy exposed—they only know very little about the lives and beliefs of their community members and receive no support or advice from the institutions they serve.

## References

Bhugra, D., ed. 1997 Psychiatry and Religion: Context, Consensus and Controversies. London: Routledge.

Birdwell, J., and M. Littler 2012 Faithful Citizens: "Why Those Who Do God, Do Good . . .". London: Demos.

Bloch, M. 1992 Prey into Hunter. Cambridge: Cambridge University Press.

Bloch, M., and J. Parry, eds. 1982 Death and the Regeneration of Life. Cambridge: Cambridge University Press.

Cole, E., G. Leavey, M. King, E. Johnson-Sabine, and A. Hoar 1995 Pathways to Care for Patients with a First Episode of Psychosis: A Comparison of Ethnic Groups. British Journal of Psychiatry 167:770–776.

Davies, D. 2002 Death, Ritual and Belief. New York: Continuum.

Domino, G. 1990 Clergy's Knowledge of Psychopathology. Journal of Psychology and Theology 18:32–39.

Durkheim, É. 1897 Suicide: A Study in Sociology. New York: Free Press.

Leavey, G. 2008 UK Clergy and People in Mental Distress: Community and Patterns of Pastoral Care. Transcultural Psychiatry 45:79–104.

Leavey, G., K. Loewenthal, and M. King 2007 Challenges to Sanctuary: The Clergy as a Resource for Mental Health Care in the Community. Social Science and Medicine 65:548–559.

Leavey, G., T. Guvenir, S. Haase, and S. Dein 2007 Finding Help: Turkish Speaking Refugees and Migrants with a History of Psychosis. Transcultural Psychiatry 44:258–274.

Leavey, G., and M. King 2007 The Devil Is in the Detail: Partnerships between Psychiatry and Faith-Based Organisations. British Journal of Psychiatry 191:97–98.

Leavey, G., J. Rondon, and P. McBride 2011 Between Compassion and Condemnation: A Qualitative Study of Clergy Views on Suicide in Northern Ireland. Mental Health, Religion & Culture 14:65–74.

Leavey, G., J. Rondon, K. Radford, M. Fawcett, N. B. O'Hagan, and P. McBride, eds. 2008 Dealing with Suicide: The Needs of Clergy in Providing Pastoral Care. Belfast: Northern Ireland Association for Mental Health.

Louden, S. H., and L. J. Francis, eds. 2003 The Naked Parish Priest: What Priests Really Think They're Doing. London: Continuum.

Mason, K., P. Polischuk, R. Pendleton, E. Bousa, R. Good, and J. D. Wines 2011 Clergy Referral of Suicidal Individuals: A Qualitative Study. Journal of Pastoral Care Counselling 65:1–11.

Mayers, C., G. Leavey, C. Vallianatou, and C. Barker 2007 How Clients with Religious or Spiritual Beliefs Experience Psychological Help-Seeking and Therapy: A Qualitative Study. Clinical Psychology and Psychotherapy 14:317–327.

McCabe, R., and S. Priebe 2004 Explanatory Models of Illness in Schizophrenia: Comparison of Four Ethnic Groups. British Journal of Psychiatry 185:25–30.

Prochaska, F. 2006 Christianity and Social Service in Modern Britain: The Disinherited Spirit. Oxford: Oxford University Press.

Stack, S. 2000 Suicide: A 15-Year Review of the Sociological Literature. Part II: Modernization and Social Integration Perspectives. Suicide and Life-Threatening Behavior 30:163–176.

Stark, R., and W. S. Bainbridge, eds. 2002 The Future of Religion: Secularisation, Revival and Cult Formation. Berkeley: University of California Press.

Taylor, C. 2008 A Secular Age. Boston: Harvard University Press.

Wang, P. S., P. A. Berglund, and R. C. Kessler 2003 Patterns and Correlates of Contacting Clergy for Mental Disorders in the United States. Health Services Research 38:647–673.

Weaver, A. J. 1995 Has There Been a Failure to Prepare and Support Parish-Based Clergy in Their Role as Frontline Community Mental Health Workers. Journal of Pastoral Care 49:129–147.

Weaver, A. J., K. J. Flannelly, D. B. Larson, C. L. Stapelton, and H. G. Koenig 2002 Mental Health Issues among Clergy and Other Religious Professionals: A Review of Research. Journal of Pastoral Care Counseling 56:393–403.

Wiesenfeld, A. R., and H. M. Weis 1979 Hairdressers and Helping: Influencing the Behavior of Informal Caregivers. Professional Psychology 10:786–792.

## Chapter 6

## Psychiatry and the Sweat Lodge: Therapeutic Resources for Native American Adolescents[1]

*Thomas J. Csordas*

### Introduction

In any community, the repertoire of therapeutic modalities available for the treatment of mental illness can be considered a reservoir of cultural resources that can be brought to bear in situations of serious emotional, cognitive and behavioral disturbance. Conceived in this way, conventional Western or biomedical psychiatry includes resources consisting of various forms of psychotherapy for individuals, families or groups, and a broad array of psychopharmacological agents. Outside the domain of conventional psychotherapy and psychopharmacology, an additional reservoir of therapeutic resources exists in the form of indigenous, folk, spiritual and ritual healing modalities.

In this context, we must note that it has only been since the middle of the last century that anthropologists and transcultural psychiatrists began to take traditional, folk, religious or indigenous healing practices seriously. Prior to that period, scholars of sound mind were as likely to regard these practices as superstitious hocus-pocus as to grant them legitimacy as forms of healing, and as likely to regard practitioners as pathologically afflicted as to recognize them as important contributors to their communities. Eventually scholars began to interpret religious healing by analogy with psychotherapy (Kiev 1963; Bourguignon 1976; Kleinman 1980; Frank and Frank 1993; Csordas and Lewton 1998).

A profound and definitive turning point was reached with the publication by Jerome Frank of *Persuasion and Healing*. Over three editions published in 1961, 1974 and 1993, Frank's work transformed the contemporary understanding of the relation between culture and psychotherapy,

---

[1] Research for this chapter was supported by the National Institute of Mental Health Grant 1 RO1 MH071781.

and prompted us to develop an expanded understanding of psychotherapy as a human endeavor not limited to Euro-American societies (Frank and Frank 1993). Frank directed our attention to the task of developing the psychotherapy analogy into a truly comparative theory of psychotherapy by identifying its least common denominator in the manner in which interpersonal stress is central to affliction, in the importance of the assumptive world that underlies therapeutic practices, in the way all forms of healing address an underlying state of demoralization, in the relevance of myth and ritual across all forms of psychotherapy and in the manner in which all these forms of healing have to do with rhetoric, hermeneutics and the transformation of meaning.

Frank regretted not having updated his chapters on religious healing for the third edition of his book, but his intellectual legacy is the condition of possibility for the new cross-cultural psychiatry developed by Arthur Kleinman (1980, 1988) and others. From a clinical standpoint, European ethnopsychiatry and North American clinics specializing in the treatment of ethnic/immigrant populations have been present since the 1960s and 1970s. More recently there has been a movement toward multicultural counseling and integrative medicine in which traditional healers are integrated into clinical treatment programs. In some cases conventional mental health professionals have received training in complementary and alternative medicine (Hager 2001; Moodley and West 2005; Johannsen and Lazar 2005; Waldram 2015).

Some of those concerned with cultural issues in counseling and psychotherapy have begun to move beyond notions of multiculturalism and cultural competency that despite the best of intentions often reduce culture to a series of formulae and seek to define competence in the form of a recipe. In the first place this shift is an attempt to get the "big picture" of diversity across the many forms of healing through history and across cultures that can justifiably fall under the umbrella of the psychotherapy analogy. This aspect of the work contributes to the broad aim of developing a comparative theory of psychotherapy. Secondly, in a variety of ways it addresses the relations among these different forms of healing in practice. In a pragmatic sense scholars ask about the ways ritual healing and psychotherapy can be integrated or used to complement each other, but also consider the possible role of spirituality in psychotherapy per se. If ritual healing is a form of psychotherapy, is psychotherapy also inherently a ritual? If certain forms of prayer can be considered to be psychotherapy, can psychotherapy legitimately include prayer as one of its therapeutic techniques?

In sum, this movement is about expanding the cultural horizons of counseling and psychotherapy. This is not an optional enterprise undertaken for the sake of allowing practitioners to deepen their professional satisfaction or enhance their ability to reflect on what psychotherapy means to them. In this historical epoch of globalization and constant flow of populations, few therapists today will go through a career in which they do not encounter patients who have recourse to ethnic or religious traditions of healing in addition to counseling or psychotherapy. Therefore the movement is necessary not because psychotherapy can be conceived broadly, but because of the world in which we live and the challenges it presents.

## The Adolescent Care Unit

This paper describes a unique circumstance in which indigenous therapeutic resources (Csordas 2000, 2002) are integrated with resources of conventional psychiatry in an inpatient psychiatric unit specializing in the treatment of American Indian adolescents. In the spring of 1990, as part of plans for the construction of a new facility to replace the aging Fort Defiance Indian Hospital (FDIH), the regional Office of Program Planning and Development of the Indian Health Service submitted to its Washington headquarters an appeal to include a 20-bed inpatient mental health unit to serve adolescents aged 12–18. Based on nationwide figures and the statement that 27 percent of the local tribal population was within the adolescent age range, the authors of the justification estimated that there were between 200 and 600 adolescents in need of intensive care in the local IHS service unit, and between 1,500 and 4,000 in need of intensive care across the entire reservation. The entire tribal population at the time was 180,102, of whom 96 percent were American Indian, and adolescents aged 12–18 numbered 22,305 or 15 percent of the reservation population.

Risk factors cited in the planning document included high poverty rates, child neglect and abuse, high proportions of teenage mothers, high rates of alcohol abuse, exposure to the suicides of others and cultural alienation. Of the most common problems reported by regional IHS Mental

Health branches, depression was most common, along with anxiety, hallucinations, delusions, alcohol misuse, school behavior problems, suicide attempts, adult-child relations and child neglect/abuse. A 13-bed adult mental health ward at the nearby off-reservation Indian Medical Center was the only IHS resource for reservation youth. Two tribally operated units on the reservation are both restricted to treatment of juvenile substance abuse. Aside from these, the only residential or inpatient care required patients to be sent to off-reservation facilities. In addition to the serious shortage in availability of adolescent inpatient treatment, the overall situation was characterized by an absence in the continuum of care (between acute and long-term hospitalization) of both adequate outpatient programs and subacute limited-term hospitalization. Proponents of the unit deplored the circumstance in which tribal youth in need of residential treatment had at times been sent to facilities as far away from their reservation in the western United States as Maine.

The unit finally approved held 20 beds; it was intended to be a regional facility serving several neighboring tribes. It was opened in October 2005 as a day treatment hospital because inadequate staffing precluded inpatient operation at first. The first inpatients were admitted in April 2006 and the patient cohort in any week typically averaged about ten adolescents, both boys and girls. After about a year the admission model was adapted to a cohort concept to remedy a problem perceived with integrating patients at random times and to allow a group of peers to go through the same therapeutic process and bond among themselves as they did so. Although in principle any member of a federally recognized tribe can be admitted to any IHS facility, and although youth from neighboring tribes constitute a proportion of patients, most available beds are filled with adolescents from communities not far from the hospital. Patients are admitted to the unit on the criteria that they must have a DSM-IV Axis 1 disorder as their primary diagnosis. Mental retardation, substance abuse and personality disorders were excluded as primary diagnoses, though comorbidity with these disorders does not preclude admission.

**Modes of Treatment: Psychiatry and the Sweat Lodge**

The Adolescent Care Unit (ACU) explicitly integrates conventional psychiatry and traditional ritual treatment. However, this is not an integration

## Psychiatry and the Sweat Lodge

of two equal systems. Hospital administrators emphasize that insofar as the unit is a medical facility, psychiatry is the authoritative discipline and therefore exercises priority in diagnostic and treatment decisions. It is also the case that conventional health care professionals vastly outnumber representatives of traditional ritual healing. Of 36 staff members including a psychiatrist, psychologist, social workers, nurses, educators, mental health technicians and clerical workers, only one bears the formal title of traditional practitioner.

On the other hand, 25 of the 36 staff members are ethnically indigenous. These include all the social workers, who serve as primary therapists for the patients, and all the mental health technicians, who spend the greatest proportion of time in direct contact with patients managing their behavior and activities during the course of each day. This lends a characteristically local sensibility to the interpersonal environment on the unit. Moreover, individual Indian staff members express different degrees of conformity with tribal cultural values and practices in their personal styles and—not necessarily the same thing—in their endorsement of traditional therapeutic ideals on the unit. This ranges from those who appear more committed to their training as Western-style mental health professionals to those who themselves have some expertise in traditional healing practices. To complicate matters somewhat, not all of the latter appear in all cases to endorse the approach of the one staff member who officially bears the professional title of traditional practitioner.

The interaction of Indian and Anglo (i.e., Euro-American) sensibilities was evident from the outset of the ACU's operation. Although the adolescent wing was built in the shape of a traditional six-sided hogan explicitly to house a unit for adolescents, for a short time before the unit was opened it was used as an elderly care ward. This proved to be inauspicious, because insofar as the indigenous culture holds that the dead are spiritually dangerous in the form of ghosts, the inevitable deaths on such a ward rendered the hopefully fresh adolescent unit in need of spiritual decontamination even before it opened. Efforts to remedy the situation were partially compromised in that the necessary traditional prayers should have been accompanied by the burning of sweet grass so that its cleansing smoke could spread through the unit, and regulations prohibited anything burning inside a federally regulated hospital facility. In another instance when the unit was already in operation, a period of high tension between the Indian staff and an Anglo clinician was marked by a number of Indian staff members coming to work wearing a kind of amulet usually associated with protection from ambient forces of witchcraft.

A wide range of treatment modalities and activities are employed in the ACU, and these can be distinguished as either conventional psychiatric or traditional ritual.

From the psychiatric side, patients in this facility are treated with individual psychotherapy or counseling, as well as with group therapy. Dialectical behavioral therapy (an elaboration of cognitive behavioral therapy) and its associated social/coping skills training are favored by some of the therapists, while others prefer a more globally nurturant/supportive therapy that may be called loosely psychodynamic. Psychopharmacology is an evident component of the treatment program, though not all patients are medicated, and a few are already on psychiatric medication when admitted. Once a week (in additional to regular evening visiting hours) a "family day" is designated in which family therapy sessions are held and psychoeducational training for parents is conducted. In addition to classes for academic work, students engage in a classroom-like art therapy session. Field trips that allow the patients to go as a group outside the hospital became a feature of the treatment program about six months after inpatients began to be admitted; these include hikes and excursions to a fitness center operated by the Indian Health Service.

From the indigenous side, young patients are treated with what may be called an identity therapy. By identity therapy I mean that the traditional practitioner's activities are oriented by the more or less explicit principle that knowing who one is as a tribal member will inherently foster health and well-being. More specifically, it means that understanding what it is to become and to comport oneself as an adult man or woman in the traditional way is essential to a healthy life. In addition to academic classes conducted by teaching staff, the traditional practitioner conducts a class on tradition and culture, with emphasis on knowledge of clan identity, myth and cosmology. According to tribal tradition, at dawn every morning each person should run in the direction of the sunrise and then home again to strengthen oneself and show oneself to the deities. The practice of morning running is incorporated into the ACU routine, even though it consists of running laps around the unit's walled courtyard.

*Psychiatry and the Sweat Lodge*

Also prominent on the ACU is a blessing ceremony each morning. Patients and some staff members gather in the walled courtyard outside the unit and stand in a circle around a small brazier into which the traditional practitioner places cedar to produce smoke. Participants sing a traditional ceremonial song, which has become known informally as the "ACU theme song," while one of the young patients is given an eagle feather fan with which he or she fans smoke onto each participant as a form of blessing. Each patient is invited to speak to the group, with words that usually consist of a simple exhortation to self and peers to think positively and have a good day, respecting one another and cooperating with staff members. Occasionally a patient will make a much more emotional or personally relevant statement, such that this brief 15 minute event can have more than a simple orienting effect on the course of the day. Staff members also occasionally make encouraging statements during the blessing ceremony. While those in the circle take turns speaking, each person silently steps toward the brazier and blesses himself or herself with cedar smoke.

On the day of each patient's discharge from the ACU, the family is invited to attend a ceremony that includes a "talking circle." Chairs are arranged in a large circle, and the traditional practitioner passes an eagle feather around the circle. While each participant holds the feather, he or she speaks words of personal acknowledgement and good wishes for the future to the departing patient, and the patient in turn speaks to each of the participants in the circle. Finally, and considered integral to treatment on the ACU, a patient may also be granted a leave of absence for one or several days to participate in a healing ceremony that may be recommended by the traditional practitioner or requested by the patient's family.

Perhaps the most prominent traditional feature of the therapeutic culture being developed on the ACU is the sweat lodge ceremony, and I will describe it in somewhat more detail. The sweat lodge ceremony is an indigenous North American practice used by a variety of tribes as both a means of initiation for young people and a technique of purification for adults. The traditional sweat lodge is a small earthen structure typically large enough for two people. Today tribal members often use a somewhat larger dome-shaped structure constructed in Plains Indian style by placing tarps or blankets over a wooden frame of bent saplings and comfortably

133

seating up to 20 participants. The local Indian Health Service Hospital maintains a site on a high ridge about two miles from the hospital where one small traditional and two of the larger sweat lodges have been constructed, one for use by men and one by women. One afternoon per week a sweat ceremony is held for male hospital employees, educators and occasional guests, and on another afternoon a women's sweat is held. The ACU now also uses this site for a weekly boys' sweat led by the traditional practitioner, and a girls' sweat led by a senior woman who works as a mental health technician on the ACU. Staff members who support the traditional healing component also attend. Depending on his assessment of personal needs and his traditional diagnosis, the traditional practitioner may also conduct private sweat lodge ceremonies for individual patients.

In preparation for the ceremony, a large fire is built and rocks are placed in the fire to heat for several hours, supervised by the traditional practitioner. Young people arrive from the ACU in a van accompanied by technicians. Hot rocks are placed in a pit at the center of the lodge, and participants enter, seating themselves around the circumference of the lodge with the traditional practitioner at the west, directly opposite the east-facing door. A flap of blankets is folded down over the door, and the ceremony begins. It consists of singing and praying in the indigenous language, teaching by the traditional practitioner about cultural values and the process of growing into an adult, and speaking; the young patients are encouraged to talk about their troubles and what they hope to accomplish in their treatment, while the adults speak words of encouragement and exhortation.

The traditional practitioner places cedar on the hot rocks to produce smoke, which participants fan onto their bodies as a blessing. He periodically splashes water prepared with sacred herbs onto the rocks to create a powerfully hot steam that causes participants to sweat profusely. After a period of time the door flap is opened and participants may choose to go outside where they can drink water and partake of an herbal tea that has purgative effects if consumed in sufficient quantity. The flap may also be opened to allow fresh and cool air to enter any time a participant in danger of being overwhelmed by the heat calls out the phrase "All my ancestors!" In a complete sweat ceremony, participants enter the lodge four times, with additional hot rocks being added for each round. In the ACU sweat lodge, often during the third round a pipe is passed so participants can smoke a kind of tobacco composed of a mixture of plants gathered from the tribe's sacred mountains. The traditional practitioner emphasizes that this sacred mountain tobacco is a remedy for dependence on marijuana, which many of the adolescent patients acknowledge using.

In addition to individual variation in how the leader of a sweat conducts the ceremony, gender differences exist in practice. Comparing my experience with that of my colleague and research collaborator Janis Jenkins, the boys' sweat appears to be more strongly didactic and oriented toward each patient acknowledging his problem and intent to overcome it, while the girls' sweat appears to emphasize narration of life experience and concern for the welfare of kin. In general, however, we can understand it to work simultaneously on several levels. It is a technique of the body in which heat, herbal tea, water, sound, darkness and smoke are used to cleanse and open the being of the participants. It is a form of group therapy in which participants can feel safe to expose their fears, traumas, failings and desires, as well as to experience the solidarity and support of treatment staff and patient peers, and to allow for the safe expression of interpersonal tension that might exist among them. It is also a critical site of identity therapy, in which the rocks are described as grandfathers who will share their wisdom, the "enfolding darkness" within the sweat lodge is described as a maternal presence that constructs the sweat lodge as a womb in which participants are safe and secure, and into which the traditional deities are invited as fellow participants and protectors. The teachings range from the elevated myth of the origin of the sweat lodge itself as the first structure created upon emergence of humans into the present world, to the most concrete injunction of bodily self-control that one must refrain from passing gas in the sweat lodge lest as a result participants develop migraine headaches.

The traditional practitioner told of taking one of these boys into the sweat lodge and learning that he was hearing voices. He explicitly noted that this would be called schizophrenia from the standpoint of psychiatry, but insisted it was not. In the lodge he told the boy to close his eyes even though it was dark. He asked the boy what he saw and the boy responded that he saw his aunt telling him to misbehave and saying that it was time for him to get up and go with her. The aunt was a ghost, and they confronted her together, the boy saying this is where I live and I want to stay.

She cried, but ended up smiling and eventually floated out of the sweat lodge. In these ceremonies participants take several breaks until they have gone into the lodge for four "rounds" of sweating and praying. In another round during this session, the boy's deceased cousin came and sat between them, laughing. Again they succeeded in getting the spirit to depart, and in the aftermath the boy became, in the view of the healer, a normal young man participating in his treatment. In other words, the normality achieved was not a cure in lieu of psychiatric care, but a normality within treatment and allowing the young man to accept and respond to that treatment.

**Resourceful Intersections**

It would be a mistake to conclude that conventional psychiatric and traditional ritual treatment modalities are simply two culturally distinct sets of practices that coexist in a mechanical, unprogrammed juxtaposition. The ideal of integration is played out on more than one level, even if at times implicitly. On the pragmatic level of everyday clinical practice, working across cultural systems is merely one challenge among the difficulties of working as an integrated treatment team and communicating insights across different clinical specialties. On the conceptual level of therapeutic logic, there are ways in which the various resources mobilized intersect and ways in which they contradict. Perhaps the most obvious intersection is that between the traditional emphasis on keeping inpatients closely connected with their families by offering treatment in this on-reservation facility, and the clinical emphasis on family therapy and psychoeducational activities during the weekly "family day."

From a psychiatric standpoint, patients are expected to progress through a series of levels from admission to discharge by achieving specific behavioral and interpersonal goals. At the same time, these levels are conceptualized in indigenous cultural terms insofar as there are four of them (four being a sacred number) that are coded in traditional colors (black, blue, yellow, white) to represent the four phases of the creation or emergence myth and a sequence that moves from "protection" of the spiritually vulnerable child on admission to "leadership" that is expected of the child engaged in his or her healing process on discharge. Finally, the ceremony marking the discharge of each patient includes both a Western-derived presentation of self and personal growth typically in the form of a collage or poetry presentation, and the Native American talking circle, which integrates the voice of the individual speaker symbolized by the eagle feather he or she holds with the strength of the social collectivity symbolized by the circle of participants of which he or she is a part.

At the same time, cultural clashes can occur when resources are differently valued. Psychopharmacological agents are prescribed for some patients, but some of the traditional Indian staff are staunchly opposed to any intervention by means of Western psychiatric medication, arguing that all they do is make patients sleepy and muddleheaded when what is needed instead is clarity and "straightening" of thought. These individuals insist instead on the value of traditional herbal remedies, which are disallowed for fear of negative interaction with Western medications and the possibility of allergic reaction to plants with unknown chemical content. In the domain of psychotherapy, some staff strongly favor therapy that is primarily nurturing and supportive while others favor therapy based on active intervention. Likewise, some insist that therapy should emphasize the positive and focus on the future, while others cite the need to resolve the harmful effects of past experiences. These disagreements in part map onto a cultural difference between the indigenous understanding that thinking about negative things brings them about or increases their power, and the Euro-American understanding that confronting negative things resolves them or decreases their power. Thus differing definitions of what it means to "think positively" can be quite consequential across cultures.

In the diagnostic domain, incommensurability is often in the air, with traditional and psychiatric understandings of causality in tension. A vivid instance arose in a case conference, the regularly scheduled meeting during which staff members reviewed and discussed the situations of individual patients. After each of the other staff members had weighed in on the case of a particular girl, the traditional practitioner proposed that her problems originated in utero when her mother witnessed an eclipse, thus exposing her to a dangerous and pathogenic spiritual influence. Silence ensued, and the implications of this hypothesis were not explored. To be sure, there was an element of challenge and defiance, perhaps of intentional provocation as well, in the traditional practitioner's analysis. Yet this could have been an opportunity to bridge cultural idioms if the mother's violation of a cultural taboo against looking at an eclipse while pregnant was understood as a sign of maternal irresponsibility, lack of being raised with proper values, or callous neglect that resulted in deficient parenting and hence the troubled state of the adolescent girl under consideration. In other words, rather than appearing to other clinical staff as a conversation-stopping magical or even superstitious attribution of pathogenic influence to the eclipse, it could have become the occasion for reconciling two ways of thinking about the importance of parental influence in the cultural context where a particular cultural prohibition was a synecdoche of an entire fabric of values related to health and well-being.

A different kind of intersection appears at the level of understanding how the conventional psychiatric and traditional ritual systems of therapeutic resources engage bodily experience. There was a time in anthropology when it was conceivable to assert that one dimension within the contrast between indigenous and industrial societies was that the former were more sensual and the latter more cerebral. Such a position is equally beholden to an invidious distinction between "savage and civilized" and to a conceptually burdened distinction between body and mind. Contemporary theorizing on embodiment leads us to celebrate the fact that a technique of the body is equally a social and meaning-generating phenomenon as well as a sensuous phenomenon. Moreover, we are disposed to examine the engagements of bodily experience in all societies, industrial as well as indigenous (Csordas 2002; Mascia-Lees 2011).

From this standpoint we can understand that the bodily construction of social space in the traditional way is characterized by orientation in terms of the four cardinal directions and the arrangement of individuals in a circle, as at the morning blessing, inside the sweat lodge, and in the talking circle. In the clinical way one finds the use of classrooms where patients are arranged in rows, group therapy rooms in which individuals are spread out on couches and chairs, and dyadic interactions in which patient and therapist face one another in chairs or across a table. Group therapy in the sweat lodge takes place in nurturing darkness and with multiple modes of sensory stimulation, while psychiatric group therapy takes place in full light with full visibility of facial expression and body language. Indigenous herbal remedies are natural substances, the use of which is accompanied by ritual practice and mythic rationale, and which explicitly engage the senses as with herbal teas, burning cedar and mountain tobacco. Psychopharmacological agents introduce manufactured substances into individuals with the understanding that they are biological agents intended to affect brain chemistry. The traditional emphasis on running each morning has the dual emphasis on building strength and endurance and on asserting one's presence and identity in the world before the Holy People. The clinical emphasis on physical fitness has the emphasis of increasing cardiovascular health and by extension the individual's self-esteem.

## Conclusion

The discussion presented above outlines the encounter between two culturally distinct systems of addressing the emotional distress of young Native Americans. What can be said with certainty is that the development of the Adolescent Care Unit marks an important moment in the history of mental health services for American Indians, and not only because it fills a pressing need. First, as the first inpatient mental health facility ever to exist within the Indian Health Service, the unit is unique in providing on-reservation, inpatient adolescent mental health care. Second, its treatment programs are being developed in a specific effort to achieve cultural relevance within the context of contemporary tribal society. Third, if successful it is likely to be a model for comparable programs in other Native American, ethnic or immigrant groups within the United States. In sum, it is a situation in which therapeutic resources are maximized in an effort to synthesize two significantly different traditions, the principal common feature of which is concern for the well-being and future development of young people. This synthesis is intended to create a therapeutic totality integrating these resources with respect to cognitive, sensory, emotional, biological and cultural dimensions of experience.

## References

Bourguignon, E. 1976 The Effectiveness of Religious Healing Movements. Transcultural Psychiatry 13:5–21.

Csordas, T. J. 2000 Ritual Healing in Navajo Society. Medical Anthropology Quarterly 14(4):463–475.

―――. 2002 Body/Meaning/Healing. New York, NY: Palgrave.

Csordas, T. J., and E. Lewton 1998 Practice, Performance, and Experience in Ritual Healing. Transcultural Psychiatry 35:435–512.

Frank, J., and J. Frank 1993 [1961] Persuasion and Healing: A Comparative Study of Psychotherapy. Baltimore: Johns Hopkins University Press.

Hager, M., ed. 2001 Education of Health Professionals in Complementary/Alternative Medicine. New York: Josiah Macy Jr. Foundation.

Johannsen, H., and I. Lazar, eds. 2005 Multiple Medical Realities: Patients and Healers in Biomedical, Alternative, and Traditional Medicine. New York: Berghahn Books.

Kiev, A. 1964 Magic, Faith, and Healing: Studies in Primitive Psychiatry. New York: Free Press.

Kleinman, A. 1980 Patients and Healers in the Context of Culture. Berkeley: University of California Press.

———. 1988 Rethinking Psychiatry: From Cultural Category to Personal Experience. New York: Free Press.

Mascia-Lees, F. E., ed. 2011 A Companion to the Anthropology of the Body and Embodiment. Chichester, UK: Wiley-Blackwell.

Moodley, R., and W. West, eds. 2005 Integrating Traditional Healing Practices into Counseling and Psychotherapy. Thousand Oaks, CA: Sage Publications.

Waldram, J. 2015 Revenge of the Windigo: The Construction of the Mind and Mental Health of North American Aboriginal Peoples. Toronto: University of Toronto Press.

## Chapter 7

## Leading and Misleading Religious Boundaries: Lessons from (Mental) Health-Seeking Practices in India

*Johannes Quack*

### Introduction

This article contributes to recent arguments questioning the appropriateness of focusing primarily on the boundaries between established religious traditions to make sense of the religious field in India. It is primarily based on a review of ethnographies of religious healing shrines complemented with my own research on (mental) health-seeking practices. It is asked where and to what degree religious boundaries lead people's decisions and actions within the pluralism of therapeutic offers in India and in what respect these are misleading. Answers to this question have to balance between over- and under-estimating the pervasiveness of religious boundaries, keeping in mind the religious identity politics of South Asia. It is argued that there are no conceptual tools flexible enough to make the necessary assessments. The article ends with advocating the heuristic notion of "modes of religiosities" to complement existing ways of looking at the role of religion(s) within South Asia's therapeutic pluralism.

### The Role of Religion(s) in India's Therapeutic Landscape

What is the role of religion in India's therapeutic landscape as perceived by psychiatrists on the one side and patients and their caregivers on the other? This was the main question of the research on which this article is based. It draws on an ethnographic study conducted over nine months in the psychiatric wing of an urban hospital in North India in 2010.[1] The

---

1   Since the fieldwork was primarily based in a hospital, this article employs the notion "patients" despite the fact that this term is misleading in non-biomedical healing environments. Besides participant observation, 93 self-designed

realm of "mental health" care in India includes psychiatry and psychology (as part of biomedicine, also referred to cosmopolitan, modern, English and Western medicine or allopathy in India), the learned or codified medical traditions (Ayurveda, Yoga, Unani, Siddha, and Homeopathy: AYUSH), recognized and supported largely by the Indian state alongside biomedicine, as well as the heterogeneous realm of "religious" or "folk" therapies (faith, local, symbolic, ritual healing practices).[2] Hence, as it is used here, "folk healing" serves as a residual category along with the term "healer" and it also covers those places often referred to in the literature as Traditional Healing Centers (THCs), a term which includes private homes as well as large public treatment centers.[3]

The anthropologist Murphy Halliburton, who conducted a comparative study of allopathy, Ayurveda and "religious therapies," argues that the former two healing systems have institutional histories and canons of knowledge and practice while the realm of religious therapies has to be thought of, more precisely, as three different therapies: "one that is prac-

---

questionnaires were jointly filled out with the patients and 68 semi-structured interviews were conducted in Hindi by me (in many cases accompanied by a resident doctor). The sample included 1 percent Buddhist, 2 percent Christian, 3 percent Sikhs, 15 percent Muslim and 78 percent Hindus and one man who noted "all" on the questionnaire. In all cases informed consent was given orally as well as in writing. I further draw on my research on "traditional" as well as institutionalized mental health care in India since 2005. This includes visits to different "folk healing" sites, interviews of patients, healers, psychiatrists, mental health activists, representatives of NGOs and self-help groups in Maharashtra and Delhi, as well as research on the criticism of religious healing practices in public discourse.

2 The Department of Ayurveda, Yoga & Naturopathy, Unani, Siddha and Homoeopathy (AYUSH) is part of the Indian Ministry of Health and Family Welfare. From 1995 to 2003 it was called Department of Indian Systems of Medicine and Homoeopathy (ISM&H).

3 As most of the other terms used here, the label "traditional" is problematic in various ways. On the one hand, it is primarily associated with the learned traditions of India (AYUSH) rather than with the "folk" realm. Further, it has often been noted that the distinction between modern and traditional practices is not only hierarchical but also fails to capture "modern traditions" (Pakaslahti 2009:161) and "multiple" or "alternative modernities" (e.g., Gaonkar 2001).

ticed at a Muslim mosque, another at a Hindu temple and the third at a Christian church. These therapies do share an emphasis on the role of the divine and a person's relation to the divine in healing illness" (2009:42). Such distinctions are characteristic for psychiatrists, social scientists and other scholars addressing the role of religion(s) within this medical pluralism, meaning they usually work with a standard conceptualization of the notion "religion." It is understood as a universal and generic concept that describes a distinct social realm (independent of other social realms such as science, art and politics), as consisting of various distinct types of religion (Islam, Hinduism, Christianity, etc.), with a belief in spiritual beings (non-human agencies, supernatural entities, the "divine" or the like) at its core and is sometimes distinguished from illegitimate, harmful and wrong beliefs and practices ("superstition" or "magic"). Accordingly, the realm of psychiatry and larger parts of AYUSH are generally considered to be secular, separate from religious ways to deal with (mental) health problems as they are found in the established religious traditions of South Asia.

Yet, there are other ways to conceptualize beliefs and practices attributed to the realm of religion in general and the role of religion(s) within (mental) health care in particular. In the following it will be shown that there are several reasons to question the pervasiveness of structuring the religious field in South Asia primarily along the lines of different religions such as Hinduism, Islam and Christianity. The most prominent and controversial challenge stems from studies that research the history and genealogy of the concept of "religion" on the subcontinent and how Hinduism was established as one of several "world religions." Secondly, there are anthropological descriptions of healers and traditional healing centers highlighting ambiguities when it comes to ascribing them to one of the established religious traditions. Finally, and most importantly for the argument of this paper, studies of "health-seeking behavior" show that the patients themselves often have ambivalent and changing perspectives with respect to dominant religious boundaries. Yet, most of the scholars researching these issues did not draw conceptual consequences from their observations, and none of their accounts helps to analyze, for example, why religious boundaries seem to matter less when it comes to health-seeking practices despite their great importance to people in other fields of their lives. The challenge for this article is therefore to carefully trace where and why one has to acknowledge the importance of established religious boundaries and where these boundaries seem to be of little relevance. Accordingly, the aim is not to challenge religious boundaries per se, which can be illuminating as well as obfuscating; the aim is rather to complement them with descriptive and analytical approaches that run transversely to established ways of structuring the religious field. One of these complementary approaches draws on the work of the historian of religion Ulrich Berner and distinguishes "modes of religiosities." On this basis this paper suggests the distinction between pragmatic and scholastic modes of religiosities.

## The History and Pervasiveness of "Religion" in Contemporary South Asia

The 2001 census of India[4] reported that out of a total of 1,028,610,328 Indians 80.5 percent are Hindus, 13.4 percent Muslims, 2.3 percent Christians, 1.9 percent Sikhs, 0.8 percent Buddhists, 0.4 percent Jains and 0.6 percent belong to "other religions & persuasions" (e.g., Jews, Zoroastrians and Baha'is), while 727,588 Indians (i.e., 0.1 percent) did not state their religion. The problems of such a census were debated extensively, especially in a historical perspective and with respect to the conceptualization of "Hinduism" as a religion. The Professor of Asian Studies Harjot Oberoi quotes Sir Denzil Charles Jelf Ibbetson, the British commissioner of the 1881 census in Punjab, noting that no other detail to be recorded "is so difficult to fix with exactness, or needs so much explanation and limitation before the real value of the figures can be appreciated" as religion. He continued that the

> various observances and beliefs which distinguish the followers of the several faiths in their purity are so strangely blended and intermingled, that it is often impossible to say that one prevails rather than another, or to decide in what category the people shall be classed. [Ibbetson in Oberoi 1994:9]

The difficulties mentioned by Ibbetson have not fully ceased. A document issued by the Indian Ministry of Statistics and Programme Implementation states that the issue of consistency in classifying "religion"

---

[4] Data from the 2011 census was not yet available by the time the article was submitted.

returns within the 2001 census and across the earlier censuses. In this respect the Indian Ministry speaks of a "truly daunting task" (Registrar General of India 2001).

Questions concerning the specific impact of the British census on politics of religious identity in India (Gottschalk 2011) and the general applicability of religious boundaries on the subcontinent (Schmalz and Gottschalk 2011) are part of larger controversies concerning the alleged colonial "invention" of Hinduism (Lorenzen 2006; Bloch, Keppens and Hegde 2010; King 2003). Irrespective of these scholarly debates, there are advocates of Hinduism who view it as a (world) religion comparable (and preferable) to other religions present all over India, but arguably particularly strong in the middle and upper classes. It is also unquestionable that there are many important "theological" differences between the various religions and their orthodoxies and orthopraxis; in fact, there are so many that there is no point in listing them here. Accordingly, the historians David Gilmartin and Bruce B. Lawrence describe the goal of their edited volume *Beyond Turk and Hindu* as contrarian to this discourse of bounded religious categories without, at the same time, "ignoring common sense" (2000:3). A similar point is made by the historian of religion Peter Gottschalk suggesting that Western scholars of South Asia should not rely too heavily on the distinction between religions such as Hindu and Muslim as descriptive adjectives and analytic categories while also admitting that these distinctions "are not without their use" (2000:3–4). The problem he sees is that these boundaries are often privileged to a degree that singular temporal, spatial and social maps get created, which imply that communal divisions exist for all South Asians at all times and in all contexts (for a similar argument, see Bellamy 2011:173).[5]

In line with these observations this paper aims at problematizing the general applicability of these maps and it advocates for the awareness that other maps can overlap with them, each alternately privileged according to context. But in contrast to the studies quoted above the focus here is not the historical dimension of such distinctions, but on their ambivalent

---

5   See also Baber's (2004) arguments that what appears to be a conflict rooted in the clash of religions in India (and elsewhere) often can be better understood as a specific form of "cultural racism" at work.

role in peoples' contemporary everyday life in general and their (mental) health-seeking practices in particular.

## Healers, Shrines and Health-Seeking Practices across Religious Boundaries

During several stretches of ethnographic fieldwork in India I visited different healing shrines and places that can be attributed to one of the main religions on the subcontinent. These included the Hindu Balaji Temple (Mehandipur, Rajasthan), the Christian Vineyard Workers' Church (Pune, Maharashtra) and the Muslim Mira Datar Dargah (Palanur, Gujarat). To structure the religious field only in this way is, however, questionable—in addition to the historical debates mentioned above—in at least two further respects.[6] First there are illustrative examples of healers, therapeutic practices and traditional healing centers that cannot be attributed easily to one particular religion, despite the fact that the dominant discourse emphasizing the boundaries between religions is quite widespread. Secondly, it will be discussed that the patients' decision to approach a specific kind of healer in one of these centers or related sites does not necessarily correspond to their formal religious denominations. As a matter of fact, formally Hindu patients frequently visit Muslim, Christian and other kinds of healers, which is also the case the other way round.

The first point is nicely introduced with an ethnographic vignette where a Hindu father described during an interview with a resident doctor and me the various experts he had visited with regard to the problems of his son. When the father mentioned that they had also visited "a Muslim who worships Hindu gods," he was immediately interrupted by the resident doctor who said in English to me: "This is controversial, Muslims never believe in Hindu gods." The doctor then turned to the father and added in Hindi: "What are you saying? Muslims do not believe in Hindu gods!" But the father continued unimpressed by these objections: "Well, here one has to differentiate, by caste [*jāti*] he is a Muslim saint but he worships the Hindu [goddess] Kali-Mā and the god Shiv[a]ji." The psychia-

---

6 For further studies discussing limits of religious boundaries, see Roy Burman (1996, 2002), Pandey (1993), David (2009) or Bloch, Keppens and Hegde (2010). And with respect to communities that defy clear categorization, see the study of a Muslim community performing Hindu rituals (Sax 2009).

trist just shook his head and signaled that it should not be believed what this fellow is saying. I, however, did not follow the doctor's advice since I had heard about this healer from other patients and since I knew from my own research as well as from other anthropological accounts that this healer would be no unicum.[7] In addition to this disagreement about the permeability and normativity of religious boundaries two further points need to be made with respect to this incidence: first, it is important to note that expressions like "medical pluralism" sometimes evoke situations where people easily choose among alternative forms of therapy, without stressing the implicit asymmetries that shape health-seeking practices as well as the positioning of distinct therapeutic practices against each other—as argued by Naraindas, Quack and Sax (2014) and particularly Naraindas (2014). Second, the therapeutic landscape in general is much more diverse than purported by the differentiation between biomedicine, AYUSH and "religious therapies." As part of the research, psychiatrists focusing on "past-life regression therapy" and psychologists versed in handreading techniques and "spiritual counseling" were interviewed. Further, the anthropologist Brigitte Sébastia rightly notes that while the differences between AYUSH and "religious therapies" are often difficult to assess, they seem "particularly clear to the government which discredits the second while promoting the first" (Sébastia 2009:7). Finally, there are not only Hindu *pundits*, Muslim *maulvis* and Christian pastors but also *babas*, tantrics, astrologers, gurus and other kinds of specialists versed in various religious healing techniques that often defy any kind of formal religious affiliation.

Similar points can be made not only with respect to one specific healer but also to larger pilgrimage and healing centers. During a short visit to the Muslim healing shrine or *dargāh* (royal court, tomb of a Muslim saint) of Mira Datar I observed what Helene Basu documented in her

---

[7] The anthropologist David Mandelbaum, for example, reports about a particularly impressive healer who listed a great many sources of healing power including the god Hanuman as well as a conjuror of Dacca in Bengal, a Muslim saint, the goddess who presides over cremation grounds and a spirit that dwells in a particular fruit tree (1966:1177). In the realm of healing it is not uncommon to employ a great range of religious traditions and references. Harish Naraindas speaks in this context of a "complete spiritual armory" or a *panoply* (2011:68; cf. the "Panoply of God": Ephesians 6:13).

ethnographic fieldwork, namely that a considerable amount of Hindu patients are visiting this shrine (2009:50). The shrine complex Husain Tekrī visited by the anthropologist Carla Bellamy, commonly referred to either as *dargāh* or as *rauzas* (tomb, garden), is described by her as "ambiguously Islamic" and as featuring a "hybrid geography and ritual life," consisting of many different types of Islamic memorial structures as well as "non-Muslim sacred spaces." For instance, a step well-constructed in memory of the daughter of the Prophet Muhammad, Fatima, is also "understood to be a point of access to both Hindu and Islamic figures, among them a form of Devī, or the great Hindu goddess, and the mahdī, or Islamic messiah" (2011:xix–xx). While Muslim saints' shrines can vary in various ways across the subcontinent she expounds that they all have one thing in common: they all are "places where individuals of all religious backgrounds seek healing and succor" (2011:4). Pilgrims of all religious, caste and class backgrounds recognize such shrines, according to Bellamy, as being of the same fundamental type. Hence,

> dargāh culture is properly understood as a (religious) culture in and of itself, rather than a culture that draws its forms of authority and practice from Hinduism, Islam, or a syncretic combination of the two. Rather than "Hindu" or "Muslim," Indian dargāh culture is South Asian. [Bellamy 2011:6][8]

A further way to challenge established religious boundaries emerges by looking at the actual health-seeking practices more closely from the people's perspective. If one reads the studies cited above through this lens, at least three important points have to be highlighted: first, Basu argues that in Gujarat many Muslims and Hindus share similar beliefs, as for example regarding the "discontentedness" of people who died an untimely death and come back to haunt the living, or in their interpretations of "insanity" that refer in similar ways to concepts of "impurity." For example, the oppositions between *shudh* and *ashudh*, *chutti* and *acchutti*, as well as *pak* and *napak* (all variations of the opposition between "purity"

---

8   She stresses the particularity of *dargāh* culture by arguing that "South Asian immigrants to Europe and North America do *not* habitually build shrines to Muslim saints even though they *do* build churches, mosques, temples, and *gurudwaras* (Sikh houses of worship) strongly indicates that Muslim saint shrine culture encompasses forms of religiosity, economy, legitimacy, and authority that are particular to South Asian culture" (Bellamy 2011:6)

and "impurity") have similar meanings in their respective uses by Hindu and Muslim communities (Basu 2009:53). Along similar lines, Flueckiger notes in her description of a Muslim healer that her religious practice "depends on a worldview shared across religious boundaries represented by its participants" (2006:8). Such shared beliefs result in shared practices and conceptualizations of misfortune and healing. Indeed, Bellamy goes so far as to argue that popular forms of religious expression, practice and narrative are themselves the true bridges across traditions. Pilgrims perceptions of therapeutic offers are not only shaped by their religious backgrounds, but the authority, power and effectiveness of such practices is also due to their physical nature, i.e., form rather than content facilitates cross-traditional exchange and participation (see 2011:18, 128).

Yet, to emphasize such shared beliefs and practices does not mean that the people are not aware of the differentiations between various religions. The second noteworthy point is that most, if not all, patients approaching healers within the "folk" sector are aware of the fact that it makes a difference to other people whether these healers are from their own religious community or not. During the interviews in the hospital many patients' answers revealed that there is also an implicit, "discursive" pressure on them to acknowledge orthodoxies and orthopraxis along the lines of the dominant discourse on religion, i.e., through emphasizing the differences in form and content between the major religious traditions. Take the example of a young Muslim man, Mr. Kalam (all names are pseudonyms), who was brought with an alcohol problem from a de-addiction center to the psychiatrist in a general hospital. He was not in good shape, rather nervous and spoke rapidly, explaining that his father was an alcoholic as well, that he worked as a driver and many things more. His flow of words faltered when he was asked about his health-seeking practices. It was obvious that Mr. Kalam didn't seem comfortable when speaking about the different healers he had approached. The first thing he said was that he was a Muslim and that he did not believe in "these other things." It was only later that he added that members of his family had first taken him to a Muslim and later also to a Hindu healer, who apparently turned out to offer the most effective treatment.

Bellamy rightly notes that Muslims more often than Hindus are subject to explicitly stated doctrinal injunctions against visiting the shrines of other religions, but that it would be wrong to conclude that "Muslims have no reason to visit Hindu temples" (Bellamy 2011:174). Dwyer notes with respect to the Hindu Balaji temple that Muslims come to the temple in the hope of receiving a cure from the deity (Dwyer 2003:170). All in all, Bellamy asserts, Muslim places seem to be visited more often by Hindus than the other way round. The generalizations made by Bellamy through the lens of her study of one particular place, however, have to be supplemented with studies of other "folk" healing shrines and peoples' health-seeking practices in general.

In addition to the example of Mr. Kalam, the anthropologists William Sax and Hari Bhaskar describe, for example, a healing tradition where at least half of the local patients are Muslims despite the fact that the negative energies and afflicting agents are described as *brahmarakshas* (literally a "Brahmin-demon") by the healers, who belong to the conservative Nambudiri Brahmins, otherwise known for their orthodoxy and emphasis of caste borders and ritual purity (2014). Further, Mandelbaum makes the general statement—with reference to the work of Beals (1962:47–48) and Bhowmick (1965:217–221)—that there is "a good deal of mutual use of the same local spirits by villagers of different formal faiths" (1966:1178). Mr. Kalam's case exemplifies that a religious self-conception (in his case as Muslim) and an awareness of the dominant discourse that emphasizes religious boundaries and differences does not mean that all people necessarily obey this norm, as long as there is no pressure for them to do so. This holds true for patients as well as healers (Flueckiger 2006:13).

The third observation to be made with respect to the role of religion(s) in health-seeking practices points into the opposite direction than the stress on shared beliefs and practices; it highlights otherness instead of similarities and shows that religious boundaries can be at play in unexpected ways. "These other things," mentioned by Mr. Kalam, were not considered less powerful by him, despite the fact, or probably because they did not belong to his formal religion. "These other things" were of particular attraction to him because they stood for unknown powers that apparently afflicted him. Bellamy argues that pilgrims' perception of the relationship between the healing shrine and Islamic beliefs and practices can be experienced quite differently depending on their own religious background. From the perspective of the non-Muslim pilgrims, *dargāh* culture "remains dependent upon a notion of others, and particularly religious others, as dangerous and potentially polluting" (2011:21). Indeed, the psychologist Sudhir Kakar noted in his study of the Balaji healing temple "that the Muslim seems to be the symbolic representation of the alien in the Hindu unconscious" (1982:87). This argument, however, can also be applied to Muslims visiting Hindu, Christian or Sikh places (and *vice versa*). It is quite generally held in South Asia that "supernatural" afflictions can be caused through religious transgression and "impurity" or "pollution." Other religious communities are a potential threat in this respect and given that they treat the dead differently and (therefore) improperly they are all the more likely to produce malevolent spirits causing afflictions. Because that "otherness" is a potential source of all that is out of place, it often has to be integrated into the healing process as well (see Bellamy 2011:180–184).

This means that sharing sacred spaces does not necessarily amount to the disappearance of boundaries and establishment of religious harmony and equality. Proponents of such an argumentation, e.g., the controversial social theorist and psychologist Ashis Nandy, have been criticized by Peter van der Veer, for projecting the modern, Western, liberal utopia of "multiculturalism" into a supposedly pluralistic and tolerant "folk culture" or a "popular religion" in India at the grassroots level (1994:190). Van der Veer himself noted that Hindus attribute great power to Muslim healing shrines, in relation to illness and misfortunes caused by spirits, thereby however not implying religious equality but reemphasizing otherness and impurity:

> A number of my informants told me that they see a connection between impurity of spirits and the fact that Muslim saints have power over them. Muslims appear to be close to the world of spirits and thus are able to master that world. In that sense they appear to be close to untouchables, who also can be specialists in exorcism. Thus there seems to be an incorporation of saint worship as a lower, impure practice in a Hindu worldview. [van der Veer 1994:193]

The task, here again, is to differentiate where religious boundaries do play an important role and where they do not. On the one side there are important differences between orthodox Islamic and Hindu "theologies" and "folk" religious practices. On the other hand one has to be careful not to produce a false dichotomy based on projections about egalitarian and harmonious folk religiosity. The assessment of leading and misleading religious boundaries has to highlight these tensions rather than overemphasize either side. In fact, rather than attempting to solve such tensions it can be argued that a second necessary and significant tension has to be taken into account, namely that between the relevance of religious similarities and differences versus the simple wish to get better, no matter how.

## Scholastic and Pragmatic Modes of Religiosity

All this goes to show that religious boundaries in South Asia can be questioned in various ways, through researching their genealogies, through a study of particular healers or healing places or through analyzing health-seeking practices. Yet, the fact that overemphasizing religious boundaries can be misleading in some respect does not diminish their pertinence in many other respects. The question for the remainder of the article is therefore: what follows conceptually from these observations and challenges? Which concepts are we to use in those cases where the standard ways to structure the religious field are not applicable? Gilmartin and Lawrence stress that in order to "open up the space between reductive religious orientations and mobile collective identities, one needs a new vocabulary" (2000:2). They try to do so by supplementing Marshall Hodgson's notion of Islamicate, a label for places influenced by Muslim rulers but not restricted to the practice of Islam as a religion, with that of Indic. "Both Islamicate and Indic suggest a repertoire of language and behavior, knowledge and power, that define broad cosmologies of human existence. Neither denotes simply bounded groups self-defined as Muslim or Hindu" (Gilmartin and Lawrence 2000:3). A similar focus on "collective identities" can be found in Bellamy's argument that South Asian "*dargāh* culture" offers a "view beyond the category of religion" (2011:6). She differentiates between "imagined" and "actual" communities, whereby the former are created without and the latter on the basis of personal contact with members of "other" communities (2011:173). While actual communities are often conceptualized within discourses of devotion and family, imagined communities are often religious ones. Gottschalk questions the exclusive emphasis on the division between religious identities and communities in India and proposes to look at the various ways in which individuals "somehow integrate multiple group identities into their individual identity" (Gottschalk 2000:39).[9]

All these approaches are partially helpful to answer the research question underlying the study on which this article is based: how is one to conceptualize the various roles of religion(s) in India's therapeutic landscape? It is important to note that people are in some contexts "Hindu" or "Muslim," and in other contexts they may participate in Islamicate and Indic language and behavior, so that they might become temporarily members of a more or less independent *dargāh* culture, while yet in other contexts their personal and group identities are based less on religious affiliations and more on class, caste, language, gender, profession or nation. Yet, the approaches listed above do not help to analyze the different ways people live their religiosities. Despite the valuable insights discussed so far we lack conceptual categories flexible enough to describe and analyze the behavior of people who reproduce and fortify religious boundaries in some parts of their life while they ignore and subvert these in other situations. How do we make sense, for example, of the observation that for some people otherwise important religious boundaries seem to matter less when it comes to health-seeking practices in general, particularly in the realm of mental health? Religious boundaries are often seen as incontrovertible when it comes to live cycle rituals. Interreligious marriages are a highly contentious matter in most of South Asia and funeral rituals generally take place in one's own religious community. But also many practices in everyday life reproduce the distinctions between religious traditions, as for example the places where to buy food, especially meat, are often organized along the standard religious boundaries. Against this observation is most interesting to note that when it comes to health-seeking practices—especially with respect to "those odd symptoms which provoke a rupture within normal social behavior" (Sébastia 2009:11)—otherwise important differentiations become less significant for some people. As Mandelbaum noted in a different context: "A Hindu villager who would never join in congregational prayers at a mosque will

---

9   General debates about forms of syncretism often implicitly reemphasize the distinctions between religions on the basis of theology-based orthodoxies and orthopraxis. For criticism of the concept of "syncretism" in the context of South Asia see van der Veer (1994) and Ernst and Stewart (2003).

quite readily make an offering at the tomb of a local Muslim saint and ask the spirit to cure him or his child" (1966:1178).

In order to make sense of this behavior and the related ambiguities of religious boundaries one has to emphasize two things. First, exchange patterns, especially of food and bodily substances, as well as life-cycle rituals, are at the center of many Hindu traditions and their related social hierarchies. Such arguments, on the other hand, are to be supplemented with the observations that the desire of people to get well can be so strong that they simply seek help from anybody accessible, affordable and with a certain reputation for healing-powers, not only irrespective of the differentiation between various religions but also between religious and medical approaches (Quack 2013). Also in this respect there is rich empirical data gathered by social scientists working in this field.[10] Campion and Bhugra argue, for example, that "in the time of distress, the religion of the healer in some instances can be of less significance than a relief from distressing symptoms" (1997:221). Banerjee and Roy note that in their study "the families went to the nearest healer or the best known among them in the locality. The method of treatment was not a criterion of choice" (1998:210). Yet, it is not enough to leave it at that, since there are also many people with strong desires to get better who would not approach a Muslim *dargāh* if they are Hindus or a Hindu temple if they are Muslims simply because it is a Muslim or Hindu place. This is an observation that can be made elsewhere and in other religious contexts as well, but one has to be careful not to confuse this argument with the simple observation that while established religious boundaries structure the whole life of some people, these are only of partial relevance to others. At

---

10 The few existing quantitative data addressing this question neither confirm nor question this argument. Campion and Bhugra argue that out of their sample, 90 percent of the Muslim patients did see a Muslim healer, 84 percent of Hindu patients saw a Hindu healer and 36 percent of Christian patients saw Christian healers (1997:218). They do not state, however, how many of them did see other religious healers alongside those of their own community. It is a well-documented fact that most patients frequent several healers at the same time or in succession and, therefore, the inverted interpretation of the data is interesting: It means that—despite the fact that people usually approach various healers—10 percent, 16 percent and 64 percent of the patients had never visited a healer from their own religious community.

stake is neither the opposition between strong and weak believers nor the fact that there are many ways to construct group identities which alternately include and exclude religious identities (Gottschalk 2000). What is at stake is that there are different ways to interpret and live one's religiosity, sometimes changing from one situation to the other. While the concept of religion(s) is definitely too static to assess such variations, there are few conceptual tools to describe and analyze such differences in religiosities. In addition to all the points outlined so far, in the following I will propose a heuristically fruitful reorientation of scholarly work to acknowledge that people live different modes of religiosities, more or less independent of their formal religious affiliation. Then the question arises, how to distinguish different modes of religiosity.

The approach to differentiate modes of religiosities developed here is based on the work of the historian of religion Ulrich Berner.[11] He shows that Christian theologians could take the same axiomatic stance on the truth of the Bible and end up either justifying or condemning the burning of witches in very dissimilar ways. In this respect the differentiation between religious traditions is of no use because we are talking about members of the same religion who, so goes the argument of Berner, exemplify different modes of religiosity. Berner further shows how skepticism can go along with a commitment to a religious tradition, even if often described as an enemy to religion(s), to the degree that it can be seen as a distinct mode of religiosity (Berner 2009:51). On the basis of historical case studies he differentiates between skeptic, fideistic, dogmatic and fundamentalist modes of religiosity. Berner's attempt thereby is not to provide a systematic typology of a limited set of religiosities; he does not suggest a top-down process where one is to find these modes of religiosities universally. Rather, he convincingly shows that this is the most fruitful way to make sense of his particular object of inquiry. The same can be

---

[11] It should not be confounded with the approach of Harvey Whitehouse (2004) to which Berner made an independent contribution (Berner 2004). It has also little in common with attempts to differentiate between "ways of being religious" (Cannon 1996) or similar attempts to differentiate kinds or dimensions of religiosity in the psychology of religion (for an overview and recent contribution, see Huber 2003) or religious studies, e.g., Charles Glock and Rodney Stark (1965, 1974) or Ninian Smart (1983). The difference is that Berner's approach is bottom-up rather than top-down.

said about the empirically grounded bottom-up distinction between pragmatic and scholastic modes of religiosity introduced in a previous article (Quack 2013). In contrast to Berner, however, the approach outlined here stresses that one and the same person may display different modes of religiosity in different situations.

In order to illustrate in what way my application of Berner's approach enables a more flexible assessment of the issues at stake, my distinction between a scholastic and a pragmatic mode of religiosity will be briefly summarized in the following. With respect to the assessment of health-seeking practices it provides a heuristic conceptual basis for cutting across the established ways of structuring the religious field. The scholastic mode of religiosity is characterized by an emphasis on ideological oppositions between secular medicine and religious beliefs and practices as well as differentiations between orthodoxies and orthopraxis within a given theological framework. It owes its name to the sociologist Pierre Bourdieu, who cautioned his colleagues against the "scholastic fallacy" that all people interpret the world as social scientists and theologians do, in this case by reproducing the dominant discourse on religion and emphasizing the boundaries between distinct religious traditions as well as religion on the one and secular medicine on the other side (Bourdieu 1990:384). In other words, patients with a scholastic mode of religiosity normally decide what kind of expert to approach for help roughly in accordance with the ways in which the concept of religion is generally understood in academic as well as public discourse. While several of them might have rationalized their health-seeking behavior ex-post, the question whether their problem is to be attributed to the religious or the medical realm was central to them. Accordingly, during the interviews patients with a scholastic mode of religiosity would reject any association with the folk sector if they considered their problems to be medical rather than religious. If asked about their religious beliefs and practices, they would make sure that these are within the realms of their formal religious affiliation. The display of such a "mode" is arguably more dominant in "modern" nation states.

A telling example of a patient with a scholastic mode of religiosity was Mrs. Negi, not only because she made clear that, being a Hindu, she would never mingle with the Muslim folks. Since she was illiterate and poor, the resident doctor Gupta deduced that she must be consulting primarily folk healers. When he inquired Mrs. Negi simply asked back: "Why should I, it is an illness [*bīmārī*]." Dr. Gupta asked her later a second time: "Did you get yourself 'dusted' [*jharvāyā*]¹² by somebody," but she denied it again. Since he did not believe her, as he thought that illiterate people like her always approached religious healers, he therefore raised the topic of religious treatment again. At this point Mrs. Negi became quite annoyed: "No, [I did] not [seek help] from anybody else, I never got anything like this done. Why should I get such things done when it is an illness." This goes to show that the scholastic mode of religiosity is not necessarily related to social status, education or income.

In contrast to the scholastic mode of religiosity, the mode of religiosity of another group of patients can be called "pragmatic." The Greek word *pragma* is translated by the philosopher Hans-Georg Gadamer—in a way that resonates with insights of Bourdieu—as "that within which we are entangled in the praxis of living, [. . .] that within which we are moving and with which we have to do."¹³ In such a perspective, religious actions as well as health-seeking decisions are not primarily geared towards orthodoxies and orthopraxis, but to beliefs and desires rooted in everyday life and limited by various constraints. This does not mean, however, that religious boundaries are not present at all. Yet, they are not primarily upheld on the basis of abstract doctrines. Indicative of a pragmatic mode of religiosity is that people simply narrate where they had to travel to, how much they were charged, the ways in which the situation improved, and—unfortunately very often—the painful relapses. The way in which such narrations are structured ignores differences between distinct religious traditions or the realms of science and religion as such. While the people obviously are aware of the differences between the visits to a *dargah*, a local shrine and a psychiatric OPD, these differences are of little concern to them. On the basis of the research on which this article is based it can be summarized—in contrast to the standard perspective of academics and psychiatrists—that this group of patients (alongside their

---

12 "Dusting" (*jhāṛna* or *jhāṛ-fuk*) refers to a practice where the "problem" is swept out of the body with a broom, but it is often used as an umbrella-term for all kinds of therapeutic practices and healing rituals.

13 My translation of "[D]as, worin man in der Praxis des Lebens verwickelt ist, [. . .] worin man sich bewegt und womit man es zu tun hat" (Gadamer 1985:6; for a different translation see Gadamer 2002).

families and friends) is less concerned about separations between the different realms of mental health care. The oppositions between secular and religious treatments or between different representatives of established religions are subordinate factors in their decision-making. The health-seeking practices of this group of patients clearly showed that they did not decide whom to approach for help on the basis of a difference between established religious boundaries. Rather, they tended to approach any expert available, affordable and endowed with a certain reputation (Quack 2013).

A qualitative analysis of 68 semi-structured interviews and respective questionnaires showed that around one quarter of the patients represented a scholastic mode of religiosity, about two fifth a pragmatic mode of religiosity, while the remaining patients, roughly one third, could not be assigned to any of the two. Such a quantitative assessment of the modes of religiosities has to be taken with a grain of salt given problems and biases like the discursive pressure to comply to the dominant view, as illustrated above with the reluctance of the Muslim patient, Mr. Kalam, to "admit" that he had seen a Hindu healer whom he considered to offer the most effective treatment. Moreover, there are examples of people displaying a scholastic mode of religiosity in one situation and a pragmatic stance in another. Irrespective of the difficulties to ascribe definitive figures to these groups it is obvious that the health-seeking practices of the people reveal important differences that cannot be described and analyzed by focusing only on the concept of religion as usually understood. Especially the theological distinctions between orthodoxy and orthopraxy of different religions can be unhelpful or even misleading with respect to patients with a pragmatic mode of religiosity.

One advantage of framing the issues at stake with respect to modes of religiosity is that this enables us to highlight similarities across religious boundaries as well as differences between people who formally belong to the same religious denomination. On the one hand, the same practices at the same place can be experienced and interpreted differently by different individuals of the same religion according to their mode of religiosity (Bellamy 2011:108; Skultans 1987). The ethnographic examples above show, on the other hand, that the health-seeking practices of people with different religious affiliations can be remarkably similar. Some take their decisions primarily according to pragmatic considerations and irrespective of their religious belongings. Others differentiate between medicine on the one hand and distinct religions on the other and rationalize their actions accordingly, i.e., they therefore share the same scholastic mode of religiosity even if they belong to different religious traditions. Moreover, a differentiation between modes of religiosities even allows us to describe and analyze how the same person can display different modes of religiosities in different contexts, i.e., obeying the dominant discourse in a conversation with religious authorities, doctors or researchers while acting quite differently in their everyday life. Finally, the way in which one and the same person makes sense of her health-seeking practices can shift between scholastic and pragmatic considerations. People all across the world do not necessarily follow one distinct "explanatory model" when they search for help. The elements of their experiences and interpretations often are not organized into functional systems or locked into nesting hierarchies of verbal classifications (Young 1981). The suggestion to distinguish "modes" proposed in this article helps to avoid the respective "scholastic fallacy" of over-interpretation and over-systematization (Dein 2007) and allows for a flexible assessment of different positions taken by one person in specific situations.

The difference between modes of religiosities such as the one between scholastic and pragmatic modes can of course be applied outside of India. Having said this, it has to be stressed again that in India religious identities are often communal rather than individual and this situation shapes the manifestation and display of certain modes of religiosity. The respective debates are highly politicized, which is partly related to the colonial history of India. Moreover, scholars cannot ignore their own role in this discourse. Flueckiger notes these involvements as well; apparently several Muslim audience members over the years raised vigorous objections to her research, telling her that "all this" was not "true Islam" but was rather influenced by Hindu culture (see 2006:11). Flueckiger goes on to note that she was internalizing this critique and considered to call her book *Healing at the Boundaries* only to recognize during her fieldwork that the practices she observed are not marginal at all (2006:12). On the ground and with respect to the actual religious practices of people in their everyday life traditional religious boundaries are often subverted, but the people can hardly ever fully ignore the dominant discourse. The pervasive religious identity politics that permeate the subcontinent are at play even in the most private conversations. With respect to Muslims that cross their religious boundaries, Bigelow notes that the rejection of sectarian religious identity alongside the attempt to uphold ones religious identity is particularly problematic in relation to minority religious communities, which are caught between national and local level identity politics (2004:32–33). And van der Veer emphasizes the "extent to which the discussion of Islamic syncretism in India is related to the position of Muslims in India after the partition" (1994:191). Frequent communal violence engraves religious boundaries in a horrific way. All this goes to show that any ascription of modes of religiosity has to take into account the respective "politics" associated with it in a specific context.

**Conclusion**

Historical studies emphasize that boundaries between religions have not always been as self-evident as they seem today in South Asia and elsewhere. Further, their contemporary pervasiveness might even be overemphasized because of a discursive pressure to comply with the dominant discourse on religion. In the realm of mental health, observations that cut across the standard ways to structure the religious field can be found with respect to healers and traditional healing centers as well as the health-seeking practices of many people. At the same time one has to be careful not to ignore powerful discourses that uphold these boundaries, especially with respect to religious identity politics, but also with respect to the importance of the distinctness of religious traditions for a concrete healing setting. The unknown powers of "these other things" can enhance cross-traditional health-seeking practices precisely because of the attributed differences.

Since the role of religion within the Indian mental health care system has partly been ignored by policy makers and medical representatives in India (Quack 2012), the notion of "religion" constitutes a helpful tool, leading us to shed light on some of the issues discussed above. In other respects, however, this notion can be misleading and has to be discharged, especially in cases where it is too static to allow adequate descriptions and analyses. Strict adherence to the standard discourse on "religion" can become an intellectualistic, rationalistic and elitist endeavor in the sense that theological elaborations are privileged over the concrete practices of the people. To illustrate this heuristic shift in research and theory it was shown that displaying a scholastic mode of religiosity means to comply to the dominant discourse on religion while a pragmatic mode of religiosity is rooted in people's decisions in their everyday praxis of living according to which the status and suitability of a healing expert can be assessed independent of religious denominations. This hopefully provides conceptual tools to further research the role of religion(s) within South Asia's therapeutic pluralism in particular and reflections on religious boundaries in general.

### Acknowledgements

Previous versions of this article were presented at the International Conference on Religion, Healing and Psychiatry held in Münster, Germany, from February 23–25, 2012. I am thankful to three anonymous reviewers of the *Journal for the Scientific Study of Religion* to which a previous version of this article was submitted. Further, the helpful and friendly remarks by Sandra Bärnreuther, Laila Prager, Tobias Schwörer and Anja Wagner are greatly appreciated. Special thanks go to Ahmed Nabil for proofreading the English text.

The work on this article was supported by the Cluster of Excellence "Asia and Europe in a Global Context" at Heidelberg University and a generous stipend by the Fritz Thyssen Foundation. Further, I was writing this article while working in the Emmy Noether-Project "The Diversity of Nonreligion," funded by the German Research Foundation (DFG, QU 338/1–1). Parts of this article are used in a monograph on the role of religion(s) within the Indian mental health care system. This book provides information about the methodology and the major findings of the larger research project introduced here.

### References

Baber, Z. 2004 'Race', Religion and Riots: The 'Racialization' of Communal Identity and Conflict in India. Sociology 38(4):701–718.

Banerjee, G., and S. Roy 1998 Determinants of Help-Seeking Behaviour of Families of Schizophrenic Patients Attending a Teaching Hospital in India: An Indigenous Explanatory Model. International Journal of Social Psychiatry 44(3):199–214.

Basu, H. 2009 'Schmutzige Methoden': Geisteskrank durch Besessenheit und schwarze Magie in Gujarat/Indien. *In* Un/Reinheit: Konzepte und Erfahrungsmodi im Kulturvergleich. A. Malinar and M. Voehler, eds. Pp. 47–66. München: Fink Verlag.

Beals, A. R. 1962 Gopalpur: A South Indian Village, Case Studies in Cultural Anthropology. New York: Holt, Rinehart and Winston.

Bellamy, C. 2011 The Powerful Ephemeral: Everyday Healing in an Ambiguously Islamic Place. Berkeley: University of California Press.

Berner, U. 2004 Modes of Religiosity and Types of Conversion in Medieval Europe and Modern Africa. *In* Theorizing Religions Past: Archaeology, History and Cognition. H. Whitehouse and L. H. Martin, eds. Pp. 157–172. Oxford: AltaMira.

———. 2009 Skeptizismus und Religionskritik. *In* Religion und Kritik in der Antike. U. Berner and I. Tanaseanu-Döbler, eds. Pp. 39–59. Berlin: LIT Verlag.

Bhowmick, K. P. 1965 Kasba Narayangarh: A Muslim Village. Man in India 45:201–222.

Bigelow, A. B. 2004 Sharing Saints, Shrines, and Stories: Practicing Pluralism in North India. Ph.D. dissertation, Department of Religious Studies, University of California, Santa Barbara.

Bloch, E., M. Keppens, and R. Hegde, eds 2010 Rethinking Religion in India: The Colonial Construction of Hinduism. London: Routledge.

Bourdieu, P. 1990 The Scholastic Point of View. Cultural Anthropology 5(4):380–391.

Burman, J. J. R. 1996 Hindu-Muslim Syncretism in India. Economic and Political Weekly 31(20):1211–1215.

———. 2002 Hindu-Muslim Syncretic Shrines and Communities. New Delhi: Mittal.

Campion, J., and D. Bhugra 1997 Experiences of Religious Healing in Psychiatric Patients in South India. Social Psychiatry and Psychiatric Epidemiology 32(4):215–221.

Cannon, D. S. 1996 Six Ways of Being Religious: A Framework for Comparative Studies of Religion. Belmont, CA: Wadsworth.

Dein, S. 2007 Explanatory Models and Oversystematisation in Medical Anthropology. *In* The Importance of Knowing about Not Knowing. R. Littlewood, ed. Pp. 39–53. Walnut Creek, CA: Left Coast Press.

David, A. M. 2009 Beyond Boundaries: Hindu-Christian Relationship and Basic Christian Communities. Delhi: ISPCK.

Dwyer, G. 2003 The Divine and the Demonic: Supernatural Affliction and Its Treatment in North India. London: Routledge Curzon.

Ernst, C., and T. Stewart 2003 Syncretism. *In* South Asian Folklore: An Encyclopedia. P. J. Claus, S. Diamond, and M. R. Mills, eds. Pp. 586–588. New York: Routledge.

Flueckiger, J. B. 2006 In Amma's Healing Room: Gender and Vernacular Islam in South India. Bloomington, IN: Indiana University Press.

Gadamer, H.-G. 1985 Die Griechische Philosophie und das Moderne Denken. *In* Gesammelte Werke. Vol. 6. Pp. 3–8. Tübingen: Mohr.

———. 2002 Greek Philosophy and Modern Thought. *In* The Beginning of Knowledge. H.-G. Gadamer, ed. Pp. 119–126. New York: Continuum.

Gaonkar, D. P. 2001 On Alternative Modernities. *In* Alternative Modernities. D. P. Gaonkar, ed. Pp. 1–23. Durham, NC: Duke University Press.

Gilmartin, D., and B. B. Lawrence 2000 Beyond Turk and Hindu: Rethinking Religious Identities in Islamicate South Asia. Gainesville, FL: University Press of Florida.

Glock, C. Y., and R. Stark 1965 Religion and Society in Tension. Chicago: Rand McNally.

Gottschalk, P. 2000 Beyond Hindu and Muslim: Multiple Identities in Narratives from Village India. Oxford: Oxford University Press.

———. 2011 A Science of Defining Boundaries: Classification, Categorization, and the Census of India. *In* Engaging South Asian Religions: Boundaries, Appropriations, and Resistances. M. N. Schmalz and P. Gottschalk, eds. Pp. 21–38. Albany: State University of New York Press.

Halliburton, M. 2009 Mudpacks and Prozac: Experiencing Ayurvedic, Biomedical and Religious Healing. Walnut Creek, CA: Left Coast Press.

Huber, S. 2003 Zentralität und Inhalt: Ein neues multidimensionales Messmodell der Religiosität. Opladen: Leske+Budrich.

Kakar, S. 1982 Shamans, Mystics and Doctors: A Psychological Inquiry into India and Its Healing Traditions. Boston: Beacon Press.

King, R. 2003 Orientalism and Religion: Postcolonial Theory, India and 'the Mystic East'. London: Routledge.

Lorenzen, D. N. 2006 Who Invented Hinduism: Essays on Religion in History, New Perspectives on Indian Pasts. New Delhi: Yoda Press.

Mandelbaum, D. G. 1966 Transcendental and Pragmatic Aspects of Religion. American Anthropologist 68(5):1174–1191.

Naraindas, H. 2011a Of Relics, Body Parts and Laser Beams: the German Heilpraktiker and his Ayurvedic Spa. Anthropology & Medicine 18(1):67–86.

———. 2011b My Vaidya and My Gynecologist: Agency, Authority and Risk in Quest of a Child. In Asymmetrical Conversations: Contestations, Circumventions and the Blurring of Boundaries. H. Naraindas, J. Quack, and W. Sax, eds. Pp. 118–161. New York: Berghahn.

Naraindas, H., J. Quack, and W. Sax 2014 Asymmetrical Conversations: Contestations, Circumventions and the Blurring of Boundaries. New York: Berghahn.

Oberoi, H. 1994 The Construction of Religious Boundaries: Culture, Identity and Diversity in the Sikh Tradition. Delhi: Oxford University Press.

Pakaslahti, A. 2009 Health-Seeking Behavior for Psychiatric Disorders in North India: An Exploration of Medical Pluralism. In Psychiatrists and Traditional Healers: Unwitting Partners in Global Mental Health. M. Incayawar, R. Wintrob, and L. Bouchard, eds. Pp. 149–166. London: Wiley Blackwell.

Pandey, G. 1993 Hindus and Others: The Question of Identity in India Today. New Delhi: Viking.

Quack, J. 2012 Ignorance and Utilization: Mental Health Care Outside the Purview of the Indian State. Anthropology & Medicine 19(3):277–290.

———. 2013 "What do I know?" Scholastic Fallacies and Pragmatic Religiosity in Mental Health Seeking Behaviour in India. Mental Health, Religion & Culture 16(4):403–418.

Registrar General of India 2001 Census of India 2001: Data on Religion. www.mospi.gov.in/national_data_bank/census_data_pro/Religion-2001/Introduction_2001_religion.pdf, accessed March 7, 2012.

Sax, W., and H. Bhaskar 2014 A Non-Modern Healing Practice in Kerala. *In* Asymmetrical Conversations: Contestations, Circumventions and the Blurring of Boundaries. H. Naraindas, J. Quack, and W. Sax, eds. Pp. 200–236. New York: Berghahn.

Sax, W. 2009 Religion, Possession, and the 'Hysteresis Effect': A Case Study from India. *In* Form, Macht, Differenz: Motive und Felder ethnologischen Forschens. E. Hermann, K. Klenke, and M. Dickhardt, eds. Pp. 181–189. Göttingen: Universitätsverlag.

Schmalz, M. N., and P. Gottschalk 2011 Engaging South Asian Religions: Boundaries, Appropriations, and Resistances. Albany: State University of New York Press.

Sébastia, B. 2009 Introduction: Restoring Mental Health. *In* Restoring Mental Health in India: Pluralistic Therapies and Concepts. B. Sébastia, ed. Pp. 1–26. New Delhi: Oxford University Press.

Skultans, V. 1987 The Management of Mental Illness Among Maharashtrian Families: A Case Study of a Mahanubhav Healing Temple. Man 22(4):661–679.

Smart, N. 1983 Worldviews: Crosscultural Explorations of Human Beliefs. New York: Scribner's.

Stark, R., and C. Y. Glock 1974 American Piety: The Nature of Religious Commitment. Berkeley: University of California Press.

van der Veer, P. 1994 Syncretism, Multiculturalism and the Discourse of Tolerance. *In* Syncretism/Anti-Syncretism: The Politics of Religious Synthesis. C. Stewart and R. Shaw, eds. Pp. 196–212. London: Routledge.

Whitehouse, H. 2004 Modes of Religiosity: A Cognitive Theory of Religious Transmission, Cognitive Science of Religion. Walnut Creek, CA: AltaMira.

Young, A. 1981 When Rational Men Fall Sick: An Inquiry into Some Assumptions Made by Medical Anthropologists. Culture, Medicine, and Psychiatry 5(4):317–335.

# Chapter 8

## "Doctor Sickness" or "Pastor Sickness"? Contested Domains of Healing Power in the Treatment of Mental Illness in Kintampo, Ghana

*Ursula M. Read*

### Introduction: Mental Illness as Spiritual Sickness

Many of the classic studies of illness and healing in Africa describe a "folk dichotomy" between illnesses with natural and supernatural causation (Fosu 1981:471). This distinction was presumed to inform help-seeking behavior and the selection of treatment between biomedical and traditional healers. In Twi, the most widely spoken language in Ghana, these are known respectively as *honam yadeɛ* (body/flesh illness) and *sunsum yadeɛ* (spirit illness), *sunsum* referring to the source of personality, character and intelligence, the part of the "dividual" self (Strathern 1988) which leaves the body during dreams and can be consumed by witches (Konadu 2007). Studies of traditional healing for mental illness in Ghana frequently categorized madness as *sunsum yadeɛ*, the consequence of *bayie* (witchcraft), sorcery, curses and offending ancestral spirits (Appiah-Kubi 1981; Field 1960; Mullings 1984; Ayim-Aboagye 1993; Fosu 1981). Such associations of madness with the spiritual resonated with anthropologists and transcultural psychiatrists, providing an anthropological rejoinder to biological reductionism in the categorization and treatment of mental illness. Coupled with a vision of the traditional healer as "native psychotherapist" (Field 1955) and an emphasis on the corporate nature of traditional healing (Turner 1967), the notion of madness as lying outside the physiological domain suggested hope for methods of treatment and cures grounded in cultural, social, psychological and spiritual approaches.

However with an increasing focus on those who seek treatment as much as those who provide it, such dualisms have given way to recognition of a dynamic pluralism, in which illness and its treatment are subjected to a process of "diagnostic trial and error" (Feierman 2000:321). Indeed a recognition of uncertainty around the causation of illness and a lack of systematization in approaches to healing has a long pedigree in medical anthropology, at least since Last's (1981) seminal article on "the importance of knowing about not knowing." An emphasis on pragmatic experimentation and empiricism when negotiating the pluralistic healing landscape of Africa has challenged notions of ideological purity in the use of healers and biomedicine, particularly in the treatment of chronic and recurring conditions (Whyte 2012; Feierman 2000; Stroeken 2012). Furthermore, as Feierman (2000:343) acknowledges, biomedicine and other forms of treatment impinge on each other in "power-laden ways." While public health services in Ghana struggle under the effects of the "brain drain," structural adjustment and wide disparity in the accessibility and quality of care, Pentecostal Christianity, as elsewhere in sub-Saharan Africa, has flourished as a source of authoritative knowledge and moral influence in all spheres of life, including health. The pervasive influence of Pentecostal Christianity has revivified the attribution of illness and misfortune to malign spiritual forces, framed within the Biblical cosmology of the demonic (Meyer 1999). Widespread fascination with the operation of magic and spiritual forces is also sustained through popular media including films, tabloid newspapers and television programs (Meyer 2003). The hierarchical division described by educated Ghanaians and health professionals contrasting progressive "modern" medicine with "backward" tradition is thus embedded within an "enchanted" society in which fears of occult powers such as curses, witchcraft, demonic possession and *jinn* are pervasive. Indeed such regressive forces may be seen to threaten, literally as well as metaphorically, the promise and progress of modern scientific expertise.

In this chapter I wish to highlight how, despite uncertainty in Ghana surrounding the nature and cause of mental illness among patients, their families and those who seek to treat them, the tropes of spiritual and physical illness are actively deployed in the discourse of both users and providers of treatment, including biomedical practitioners, traditional healers and Christian pastors. Such discourse is central not only in establishing therapeutic superiority among healers and attracting customers, but reflects an ongoing concern with the morality and legitimacy of healing power, whatever the vehicle through which it may manifest. Faced with the burgeoning popularity of spiritual healers and Pentecostal prophets offering miraculous cures and the presumed "ignorance" of those who use them, health workers in psychiatric services, bolstered by international mental health campaigns and funds from NGOs and donors, promote an overtly modernist counterview of mental illness as a "medical disease" with psychotropic drugs as the only genuine treatment. However for sufferers and their families such drugs, as much as traditional, Muslim or Christian treatments, often fail to bring about a permanent cure, casting doubts over the authority of healers of all persuasions. I argue that polarizing discourses, which contrast professional claims to offer the "correct" medical treatment with the ignorance of those who seek help for mental illness elsewhere, overlook family experiences of the limitations of psychiatry and the complexity of the therapeutic journeys undertaken to resolve the disruption and distress of severe mental illness. A close ethnography of help seeking for mental illness shows that such journeys are more often marked by uncertainty than by ignorance as families seek to make sense of mental illness and return the affected person to his or her social role.

This chapter draws on ethnographic research with people with mental illness and their families in the rural market town of Kintampo, Ghana, and surrounding villages over a 20-month period between 2007 and 2008. The research was conducted together with Solomon Nyame, a local psychology graduate who acted as research assistant and interpreter. Informants were identified who displayed symptoms recognized as signifying *dam*, "madness," or *adwen mu yadeɛ*, "sickness in the mind," characterized by chaotic unruly behavior (*basabasa*), disordered speech and a breakdown of social functioning, resembling what, in psychiatric terms, would be diagnosed as psychosis, mania or schizophrenia. Most had experienced episodes over at least a year, some over a much longer period. The recurring nature of the illness had a devastating impact on the sufferer and the household, leading to a costly and prolonged search for healing. During the course of fieldwork I met with over 60 people with mental illness in shrines, church compounds (commonly known as "prayer camps") and households, and conducted formal interviews relating to 42 of these, where possible with the sick person, and also with family members. I made regular visits to family homes, a shrine and three churches where people with mental illness received treatment. The shrine was an *abosomerafoɔ* (executioner) shrine, ritual sites which proliferated at the turn of the last century to combat witchcraft and sorcery (McCaskie 1981). It was established by the elderly *ɔkɔmfo* (pl. *akɔmfoɔ*), a term usually translated as "traditional healer" but which refers to one who is possessed by the "gods" (*abosom*) who instruct him (less frequently her) in the use of herbal medicines and reparative rituals. The churches are led by Pentecostal pastors who claim to have a particular healing gift bestowed by God, and who often set up prayer camps where people can stay for weeks or months to seek divine intervention through prayer, fasting and deliverance from evil spirits. Psychiatric treatment is also available primarily through the three national psychiatric hospitals which are clustered in the south of the country, but attempts at decentralization have led to some provision of mental health care through regional hospitals and community psychiatric nurses, one of whom was transferred to Kintampo during the course of fieldwork. I spent time with the psychiatric nurse on her community visits and in her clinic, as well as visiting national and regional psychiatric clinics and hospitals on several occasions.

**Hospital Medicine: The Last Port of Call?**

In discussions with health workers, researchers and NGO campaigners I would often be told that the psychiatric hospitals were the "last port of call," employed only after other sources of treatment such as prayer camps and shrines had been tried and failed. An NGO poster which featured a pastor brandishing a Bible over a cowering and chained madman urged the families of those with mental illness to "get treatment for them at the psychiatric hospitals and clinics before anywhere else." It was therefore somewhat to the surprise of myself, and also my assistant, to find that nearly all those we met with mental illness had used the psychiatric hospitals during their search for a cure. Though, as health workers reported, some had approached the hospitals only after other forms of treatment, such as traditional or Pentecostal healers, had failed, several had approached the hospital as the first port of call, inverting the "therapeutic itineraries" (Peglidou 2010) reported by health workers. Indeed such itineraries were highly heterogeneous, marked not by a linear progression through a "hierarchy of resort" (Romanucci-Ross 1969), but by *kyinkyini* (roaming around) within a marketplace of competing "powers" (Graveling 2010)—Christian, "traditional" or biomedical—in a search for the "last stop," an ultimate cure. Mariam, for example, fell ill in her last year at school. Her "mind was not there," and she began to behave strangely, claiming she could see *jinn* and setting fire to clothing. Her

Muslim family had first taken her to the hospital, then to a succession of Muslim and traditional healers, following rumors of their reputed power in treating madness. Her father told us:

Somebody will come and say: "Oh, some man is here, his medicine is very, very good," and we go there. So somebody who is there will say: "No, this place is better," then we go there too. And so we have roamed around a lot.

The term "the last stop," the call of the informal conductors ("mates") on Ghana's most popular form of transport, the ubiquitous minibus or *trotro*, underlines the search for healing as a journey with a hoped-for goal, often, as on the *trotro*, a long and torturous one. The "last stop" was often elusive with the search ending in disappointment, despite the repeated use of healers from diverse traditions at considerable effort and expense. Though such journeys were often fruitless, the distinction between diseases of the body and spiritual illnesses, or "naturalistic" and "personalistic" in Horton's (1967) terms, is most clearly recognized through such failures of treatment. In Ghana an illness which is unusually prolonged or fails to respond to treatment raises suspicions that there is "something behind it" (*biribi di akyi*). The significance of a disease's persistence in the evaluation of illness aetiology and the approach to treatment has a long history which predates the advent of biomedicine. Horton (1967:60) describes how African "native doctors" begin with a specific herbal treatment, and if the illness does not respond, try another. It is only after various treatments fail that "the suspicion will arise that 'there is something else in this sickness.'" In Ghana, the historian McCaskie writes that in the precolonial period "troubled individuals habitually took their problems to a succession of *abosom*" (1995:123), the "small gods" of the shrines.

Despite its enduring epithet as *aborɔfo duro* (foreign or white man's medicine) and well-founded concerns regarding the quality of hospital treatment, particularly in rural areas (Horton 2001), biomedicine has been incorporated into this "pluralistic political economy of belief" (McCaskie 1995:123), less as an exotic foreign import, than a "valuable cultural resource" (Whyte 1992:173). The Accra Psychiatric Hospital, "the asylum," founded in the opening years of the last century, is well known as a place where the seriously mad can be treated. As one informant said referring to "some town they call Asylum": "I know that doctors can treat that sickness very well." Trying out "hospital medicine" through "pills" or "injections" is as much a part of the process of identifying a spiritual illness as consultations with healers or pastors since the success or failure of biomedicine is an important empirical marker of the cause and nature of illness (Brodwin 1996; Feierman 1985). Suspicions of spiritual illness therefore arise in a dialectical relationship with biomedicine, reinforced particularly in chronic conditions which, by definition, cannot be cured by medical science. This emphasis on the relative therapeutic efficacy of biomedicine and other forms of healing rather than the nature and cause of an illness per se was reflected in conversations where we heard less reference to the distinction between spiritual or bodily illness than between "pastor sickness" (osɔfo yareɛ) or "hospital sickness" (asopiti yareɛ).

## "Ignorant" Villagers and "Spiritual Beliefs"

Nonetheless, despite the advent of psychiatry and the asylum, the concept of madness as a category of spiritual disease remains a powerful trope in Ghana, vividly reinforced in popular culture and the media. A recurring narrative in "Nollywood" films features a deranged and semi-naked madman or woman as the victim of witchcraft (Aina 2004; McCall 2003). For health workers such "spiritual beliefs" are widely presumed to inform decisions regarding treatment choices among the families of those with mental illness, as Pigg (1996) notes of assumptions regarding "villagers' beliefs" and the use of shamans in Nepal. An educational film on mental illness and human rights produced by the Ghana branch of an international NGO began with this quote: "In Ghana mental illness is associated with all forms of spiritual beliefs or absurd or ridiculous explanations." The discourse of "ignorant villagers" is a potent one in Ghana (Andersen 2004), invoked when contrasting rural and urban areas, and the less developed north from the south. These distinctions reference those between the primitive and civilized, modern and traditional, rooted in inter-ethnic struggles for political dominance, and colonial and missionary terminology.

Such distinctions are inadvertently reinforced in the contemporary discourse of national and international development agencies, which focus efforts to improve education and health on "less developed" areas, predominantly northern and rural. National health campaigns are often cast in terms of "awareness raising" of health conditions, their causes and treatment. In the day-to-day interactions of health staff with their patients, "ignorant" or "superstitious villagers" may be berated for delaying or discontinuing treatment and turning instead to the "fetish," "quack doctors" and "419 pastors," the last referring to Nigeria's notorious penal code for fraud to indicate pastors who enrich themselves through fraudulent claims of miraculous powers. As in the image on the NGO poster mentioned above, the discourse of ignorance and "superstitious" beliefs serves to distance the psychiatric community from the practices of Christian prayer camps and healing shrines where patients are routinely chained and often beaten and forced to go without food. The Commonwealth Human Rights Initiative, in a report exposing the abuse of people with mental illness within prayer camps, unequivocally stated the "ignorance" of those seeking healing, which it elaborated as "the lack of understanding that mental illness is a medical condition requiring medical attention and the belief that supernatural powers are the causes of mental illness."

Certainly the discourse of families was marked by ignorance, but not quite in the sense that health workers implied. Rather than holding to "spiritual beliefs," for most informants the cause of the illness was usually a matter of conjecture rather than conviction, particularly in the face of the repeated failures of various therapies, including biomedicine. This was signified by the most frequent response to enquiries as what had brought about the illness: *mentumi nhunu*, "I can't see/perceive," otherwise translated as "I can't tell." Though healers might identify a spiritual cause, such pronouncements were cast into doubt if attempts at addressing witchcraft or demon possession failed. Like Mariam's father, Stephen's father had also "roamed around," vainly seeking a cure for his son's longstanding illness. As he put it: "I took various paths but it didn't help me." Stephen's father explained how he had rejected a healer's diagnosis of witchcraft in the family since the prescribed cures did not work:

at first, the herbalist, he went to ask [the gods] and he said the sickness came from the family. The family gave the sickness to him. Before, he gave him the herbs. And I prayed over it. But still the same.

He finally concluded: "Whether he brought the thing from heaven or he took it from down here, I can't tell." Furthermore, at the shrine the focus of the ɔkɔmfo's treatment was less on divining spiritual causes than on administering the African medicine (*abibiduro*) for which he was renowned. Kwabena, a young man being treated with herbal medicine at the shrine, told us that the ɔkɔmfo had not told him anything about the cause of his mental illness:

Some people come here nowadays and he tells them where their illness is from, but as for me he did not tell me where mine comes from. All he told me is that I should take the medicine and it will stop.

The ɔkɔmfo's medicine was valued by families for its powerful sedative effect on the most disruptive symptoms of agitated or aggressive behavior or prolonged sleeplessness and was often the primary reason for choosing the shrine as a place of treatment, rather than "spiritual beliefs" or a desire for ritual interventions such as the undoing of a curse or countering witchcraft. For some Christians and Muslims avoiding active participation in the rituals of the shrine and restricting treatment to the ɔkɔmfo's herbs also enabled them to reconcile their use of traditional healers with their religious practice which forbade dabbling in such rites.

## The Ambiguity of Power

The relative efficacy of treatment, whether administered by doctors, healers or pastors, is essentially a test of power (*tumi*) whose essence is often conceived in spiritual terms as the ability to manipulate substances (medicine) to heal or to harm. The possession of *tumi* is what enables healers and pastors to perceive witchcraft or evil spirits which might cause a disease (Minkus 1980). Indeed *tumi* might similarly enable a doctor to make a diagnosis, as well as give potency to pharmaceuticals as much as herbal remedies. As with the ɔkɔmfo's herbal medicine, the sedative effect of antipsychotics such as chlorpromazine was impressive and valued by families as demonstrative of the potential power of "white man's medicine." The discourse of power therefore permeates the relationship between medical practitioners, traditional healers and Christian pastors, each seeking to demonstrate their superior knowledge and efficacy. The recurrent nature of psychosis, an illness which "goes and comes back" as one carer described it, opens the field for healers to stake their claim to bring about a potent and lasting cure. The common narrative structure of "miracle healing" in church testimonies, sermons and healing crusades is that God's power would bring about the complete cure which had evaded medical science, inverting the health workers' narrative of the hospital as the "last point of call" after all else has failed. Pastor Owusu, who led one of the churches in Kintampo which treated mental illness, explained how his method of healing—"hard" or strong prayer—was superior to both hospital medicine and traditional healing:

> What I see about it is that most of the sicknesses are not doctor sickness. It is spiritual sickness. Those which are spiritual sicknesses, you'll go to the doctor but it won't work. You will go to a herbalist. Some of the herbalists can work with spirits, but what I see about that aspect of sickness is that for spiritual sicknesses only very hard prayers can help you. Because some can heal your sickness but after a short time the illness comes back. Some of it comes like that, the spirit which is disturbing you, if you don't pray, the spirit won't leave. You will do and do, the person will never be healed. Unless you pray to remove that spirit, the person will never be well.

Yet claims to such powers could also be suspect since *tumi* is fundamentally ambiguous and could as easily originate from the Devil as from God (Gilbert 1989; Akyeampong and Obeng 1995). Power is rendered morally suspect if it is thought to have been obtained illicitly through the use of bad medicine (*juju*) or witchcraft. *Tumi* could be used to enrich oneself and bring about the downfall of one's enemies, even through inflicting madness, as the Nollywood films depicted. For many Christians the powers of the shrines are dangerous and fearful, and rumors abound of politicians whose power has been attained through esoteric rites and the use of "bad medicine." Though widely respected as "men of God," some pastors are also rumored to get their powers from *akɔmfoɔ*, as my companions suspected for two pastors we encountered when visiting the shrine. As Akyeampong notes, "the source and nature of the power used in Christian miracles in Ghana is sometimes, itself, disputed" (1996:165). Maame Grace, another pastor who worked with the mentally ill, told us that some people suspected that her impressive power over illness might be due to witchcraft: "People are surprised so sometimes people say that I use witchcraft to do it . . . At times the way the healing comes instantly surprises them."

Therefore, as with the health workers, the families of those who were mentally ill also demonstrated skepticism towards the claims of "419 pastors" and other healers. Mohammed's mother had visited several healers to little effect and referring to healers' "deceptive tricks" told us: "You know herbalists, they will tell you what will get them money." Media stories frequently unmasked pastors who had grown fabulously wealthy through charging their customers, or offered women healing in exchange for sexual favors or bathing naked in "holy water." However, operating outside a hierarchy of regard as much as resort, patients and their families extended such skepticism to biomedicine. Like traditional healers and healing pastors, hospital medicine for many had little lasting effect in achieving the desired cure. Psychotropic medicines, while recognized as "powerful" in their sedative effects, could be appraised as in fact "too strong," causing unpleasant and incapacitating effects such as stiffness, protruding tongue, salivation, excessive sleeping and eating and a prolonged feeling of drowsiness and weakness (Read 2012). A wariness towards pharmaceuticals is perhaps not surprising where outdated supplies and incorrect prescriptions, including excessively high doses, are not uncommon. However the side effects of psychotropic medication, in particular the sedating effect, were especially troubling where strength (*wɔ ahoɔden*) is synonymous with health. Medicines of all kinds, including herbal tonics and alcoholic bitters, are most valued for their "power" in restoring bodily vigor and vitality, including sexual potency. A strong body is needed for work, particularly farming, the most common occupation in Kintampo, as well as household chores and childcare, all of which require early rising and hard physical labor. The lassitude which could result from severe mental illness (described in medical terminology as "negative" symptoms or the "deficit syndrome") meant that those affected were often unable to contribute to household productivity and were sometimes castigated as "lazy."

For patients and their families therefore the weakness induced by psychopharmaceuticals indicated a powerful effect in the wrong direction when the desired effect was less lethargy and greater integration into productive family life. Even where signs of madness such as speaking to oneself or aggressive or agitated behavior might be reduced, in the long term it was the effect of medication on productivity which was most indicative of their power. The sedative effect of antipsychotics as well as the unpleasant effects on the body led many to discontinue taking it. Kofi was typical of many who had "roamed around" seeking treatment, first from the psychiatric hospital where he had run away, then from shrines and churches, all without lasting effect. Kofi now lived with his mother and sister and had stopped washing, stripped naked and attempted to attack family members with an iron bar. As a consequence he was shackled and locked in a room. After a visit from the community psychiatric nurse he started taking antipsychotic medication which was given to him by his mother. After some weeks Kofi recovered sufficiently to be released from the shackles, his aggression subsided and he began to interact with family members. Having seen this improvement Kofi's family was keen for him to continue taking the hospital medicine, but he refused, preferring to visit a local church where he engaged in prayer and fasting and helped farm the pastor's land. When we visited we would find Kofi, disheveled and unwashed, working on the family land around his home. He told us he did not want to take the nurse's medicine because it made him feel sleepy and unable to work. Similarly Comfort, who we met at a prayer camp, told us how she had been to the hospital and been given medication but quickly discontinued: "When I took it the first day, I slept deeply. And all my body became very weak. So I said I won't take it anymore." If symptoms returned when the drugs were discontinued, this further questioned their therapeutic power.

Campaigns by the international psychiatric community which aim to standardize the "evidence-based" treatment of psychosis worldwide and increase access to psychotropic drugs (Patel and Thornicroft 2009) have allowed little room for consideration of such difficulties. The plentiful evidence that many patients worldwide discontinue treatment with psychotropic drugs for similar reasons (Lewis and Lieberman 2008) is scarcely acknowledged in discussions regarding the "scaling up" of mental health treatment along the lines of mental health services in high-income countries. In Ghana, the limited efficacy of psychiatric treatment is usually attributed by health workers to failings or ignorance on the part of families or patients who do not adhere to medical prescriptions and do not return for medication supplies. Though additional medication is routinely prescribed to counteract the side effects of antipsychotics, there was limited discussion with patients and families regarding their impact, and there were virtually no resources for psychological or social interventions which could act as complementary or alternative treatments. Despite the potential efficacy of psychological or family-based treatments for psychosis in settings like Ghana, where material and human resources and expertise are limited, the power of hospital medicine is more often distilled to the technology of the "pill" (Jain and Jadhav 2009). This leaves aside the complex psychosocial context of mental illness and reinforces the role of other healers in addressing such concerns.

## Madness and Morality

Nonetheless it is clear that while promoting an explicitly scientific view of mental illness to their patients and their families, most of Ghana's health professionals share their spiritual beliefs, though many would draw the line at visiting a shrine. Though one could argue that such beliefs are "bracketed out" during psychiatric practice, such bracketing is not always successful, nor does it reflect the ways in which psychiatric practice in Ghana exists in dialectical relationship with spiritual practice and belief, for both the patient and the practitioner. It was not uncommon for the relatives of those with mental illness to recall how during their search for treatment, medical practitioners had diagnosed a spiritual sickness and advised them to seek treatment elsewhere. Fatima's father described how he took his daughter to the hospital when she started behaving strangely:

When the sickness came I took her to the [Kintampo] hospital and they gave me a letter that I should take her to a specialist at Sunyani. When we went they put her head in a computer. They said there might be something in her head. The doctor said that there is nothing in the head so we should take her for African medicine. So I brought her to the [Kintampo Health Research] Centre here, and they referred me to Sunyani. I sent her there and they didn't give us any medicine. They said that they didn't see anything so it is a spiritual disease.

Gifty's mother, who I met at the shrine, told a similar story: "The first time I took her to the doctor and the doctor told me it was a spiritual sickness so I should take her to a prayer camp."

Thus the discourse of madness as a "spiritual" disease seeps out in the interstices of official practice. Though it was hard to verify the retrospective accounts of informants, conversations between the psychiatric nurse and my research assistant with whom I carried out many family visits sometimes speculated on possible spiritual or moral factors which might have brought about the illness, such as Akua, a woman being treated at

Pastor Owusu's prayer camp, whose persistent mental illness was rumored to be the consequence of her seduction of a married man. "Juju psychosis," a term used by several mental health workers, referred to madness brought on oneself through dabbling in sorcery or "bad medicine," deftly combining scientific and spiritual diagnosis. Most often, speculation centered on the role of envy in bringing down rivals through inflicting madness. Fear of the envy of others lay like a shadow under overtly friendly interactions, echoing Geschiere's (1997) description of witchcraft as "the dark side of kinship." Any modicum of success led to fears that someone might try to "bring you down," referred to with typical black humor as PHD ("pull him down"). Several of those I met with mental illness had just completed secondary school, or were about to enroll, or were near completing their studies when the illness began. Others were about to begin or had just commenced "elite" careers, such as joining the army, or were about to embark on overseas travel, or were already living overseas. All of these were evidence of potential for current or future prosperity and a privileged status, and were seen as provoking the kind of envy that might lead to attempts to bring them down. The most common mechanism to enact such envy was through *sikaduro*, literally "money medicine" but translated as "blood money," the ritual exchange of the health or sanity of another for one's own wealth or success. On an early visit to Ghana I was visited by a senior psychiatric nurse who described in detail a clear case of *sikaduro*. He recounted how he had visited the brother of a young man who had been admitted to the psychiatric hospital following a mental breakdown. The brother, he recalled, was setting up a new business and had shaved his head. The nurse immediately recognized this as evidence that the man had given his brother in exchange for his success—the shaved head was a sign of his covenant with the shrine. The nurse confronted the brother and instructed him to break his covenant: "Let your hair grow and the boy will get well." When he returned some time later he found that the man's business had closed and his brother had in turn recovered. Such interweaving of popular discourse on the moral and spiritual origins of mental illness explained the failure of biomedicine in such cases, not just for families seeking a cure, but for professionals whose attempts to treat had been unsuccessful. If those illnesses which failed to respond to hospital medicine could be categorized as having spiritual origins and thus outside the purview of biomedicine, for other disorders this left the efficacy of psychotropic drugs and the biomedical model unchallenged. The flexibility of the discourse of spiritual illness, or "something behind it," its incorporation in traditional, Christian and Muslim practice, as well as its inherent nature as ultimately "unknowable," a subject for speculation rather than certainty, ensured its continued explanatory and diagnostic utility for families and mental health professionals.

Even failures of intervention by Christian or traditional healers did not necessarily undermine the explanatory value of "spiritual illness," since the persistence or recurrence of mental illness despite treatment could be attributed, as with Akua, to a failure to confess to misdemeanors which had brought about the illness. The role of confession, an integral part of rituals of healing at the shrines and churches, illustrates the framing of mental illness as a consequence of moral weakness or transgression. Though madness brought about through sorcery, curses or witchcraft might strike an innocent victim, as with "juju psychosis" it was often viewed as "self-inflicted," or, as Pastor Owusu put it, "they get it through things they do":

Mental illness itself, there are some through a spirit they can give it to someone. They can give the mental illness to you so your mind will be confused. There are some, they get it through things that they do, for example through smoking cannabis, or smoking cigarettes. It can come through that way. There are some too where it is not cannabis and it is not cigarette, but it is in the family. They can do it to you that spiritual way. Through a spirit they can give it to you.

The pastor's statement references the polarities of mental illness as either "given" to someone, often by a jealous family member, through witchcraft, *sikaduro* or a "bought" illness (*nto yaree*) purchased at a shrine and inflicted on someone, or as brought on oneself through moral misdemeanors. Aside from the use of "bad medicine," prominent among such misdemeanors is smoking cannabis, dubbed *bonsam tawa* (Devil's tobacco) and widely viewed with strong moral disapproval. The association of madness with the use of cannabis has been seized on by medical practitioners as a case exemplar for a modern view of mental illness, allowing the moral debate on the origins of mental illness to be transplanted onto the immorality of youth, rather than taboo infraction, sorcery or witchcraft as preached at the shrines and churches. One TV program even reported "drug abuse" to be the cause of mental illness for 90 percent of male inpatients in the psychiatric hospitals. However this association of madness with cannabis serves paradoxically to reinforce a moralizing view of madness (Gureje et al. 2005), which is in turn taken up by the churches and shrines, as Pastor Owusu's statement reveals. Indeed cannabis use can itself be attributed by pastors or *akɔmfoɔ* to the influence of demons or witchcraft as the ultimate cause, as Maame Grace explained regarding the mental illness of a young man at her church:

The time . . . he rolled the wee the spirit was also there, so the moment [his friend] gave it to him and he inhaled the wee the spirit entered him. Because someone smoked wee, let's say from childhood, but up to now the person hasn't gone mad, the person hasn't had any effect, but because a spirit is involved, so the madness comes at once.

Through such interchange the moral discourse of *sunsum yadeɛ* rather than dissipating is reinvigorated, for both those who provide treatment and those who use it. The limited success of all forms of treatment including biomedicine, and the proliferation of healing churches who draw on this discourse to promise miraculous cures, pushes families on in their desperate search for the "last stop."

## Conclusion: Collaboration or Competition?

The promotion of psychiatry as the modern and scientifically validated approach to mental illness in low-income settings is often depicted as the reproduction of a hierarchically ordered system, in which the authority of biomedicine, supported by proven efficacy and powerful global networks, will gradually supplant "traditional" and ineffective local treatment. However this vision does not engage with evidence for the limitations of psychiatric intervention and continuing scientific uncertainty surrounding the causes and course of mental illness. Nor does it acknowledge the extent to which assertions of medical efficacy may be inserted into a complex terrain of competing claims to power and authority over illness and misfortune. In Ghana, despite the private speculations of individual health workers, the competition for authority over mental illness with traditional and faith healers allows little room to acknowledge uncertainty regarding the nature and causation of mental illness and the best methods of treatment. Indeed the global push to scale up treatment for mental disorders advocated by WHO and the Global Movement for Mental Health (Lancet Global Mental Health Group 2007) strives to maintain ideological coherence and standardization as evidence of universal legitimacy (Orr 2012; Béhague et al. 2009). Standardized "packages of care" based on systematic reviews of evidence aim to offer the same treatment in whatever location, subject only to "cultural adaptation" (Patel and Thornicroft 2009). Adherence to such standardized treatment formulated in international guidelines has become the yardstick by which the modernity and integrity of mental health services are measured and increasingly infiltrates the training of mental health professionals worldwide.

By contrast those who experience mental illness and embark on a search for treatment explicitly confront the uncertainty surrounding mental illness by freely transgressing the boundaries between the "traditional" and the "modern" (Hampshire and Owusu 2013), reducing the vertical hierarchy of resort to a horizontal plane of healing potential. Rather than adhering to an unchanging tradition, for "traditional" and faith healers diversification and innovation enables them to distinguish themselves as offering a unique cure, while for patients and families a plurality of options allows them to try out different therapies to find a "fit" (Halliburton 2004)—whether that be interpersonal, theological or aesthetic. The limitations of psychiatric treatment in low-income settings like Ghana are exacerbated by structural failings in health care delivery, particularly for mental illness, which jeopardize the quality of treatment. Rural clinics in particular are staffed by personnel with limited training and supplies, and treatment is largely restricted to the dispensing of medication, rather than rehabilitation or family interventions and support. Disappointed families are therefore as likely to have faith in the promises of other healers since all forms of treatment are subject to the same empirical test—will this treatment bring about a lasting cure?

Faced with the enduring popularity of traditional healers, and a shortage of personnel and other resources, the WHO and other international bodies have long called for "collaboration" in the treatment of mental illness, with hospitals providing medicine and the churches and shrines offering psychosocial and spiritual interventions (Campbell-Hall et al. 2010; Offiong 1999; Ae-Ngibise et al. 2010). However attempts to enact such collaboration can perpetuate the kind of dualism which may foreclose its potential. Calls for collaboration with traditional healers in the care of mental illness in Africa have tended to emphasize their cultural congruence with "traditional" values in addressing perceived psychological, spiritual or moral aspects of mental illness, or, as with Turner's "corporate" model (Turner 1967), their role in resolving family or community conflicts. This focus on the "traditional" in healing generally overlooks the growing influence of Christian healers and the increasing diversity and hybridization of healing practices (Hampshire and Owusu 2013). It also sets aside the use of herbal medicines which, as with the ɔkɔmfo in this study, are central to the practices of many traditional healers (Morris 2011; Stroeken 2012). The medicinal practices of traditional healers support a model of competition rather than collaboration since healers concur with psychiatrists that herbal medicines and pharmaceuticals cannot safely be taken concurrently, meaning that families must choose one or the other. The delegation of psychosocial interventions to traditional healers also maintains the concentration on pharmacology as the primary intervention of psychiatry and may perpetuate a disengagement within professional mental health services from the social and psychological implications of mental illness. Moreover, collaboration is often envisioned as a hierarchical one—the medical professionals "train" traditional healers (Ventevogel 1996) and encourage them to send those they cannot treat to the hospital. Calls for regulation and oversight to combat the use of chains, beatings and other deprivations in prayer camps and shrines can ring hollow when the psychiatric hospitals continue to offer a poor standard of care with reports of beatings, neglect and corruption (Anas 2009; Human Rights Watch 2012).

For those who use healers the desire for effective treatment overrides a need for ideological or theological coherence. True collaboration or cooperation would mean an honest engagement with the experiential knowledge of those who offer and those who use healing which moves beyond the polarizing stereotypes of traditional superstition and infallible modern science to recognize the inherent uncertainty of severe mental illness and the dilemmas of treatment. Indeed the family experience of stigmatized disorders such as mental illness often throws the stereotypes and assumptions of popular discourse into question (Dennis-Antwi et al. 2011; Ingstad 1995). This opens an opportunity to work creatively with families to seek solutions which attend to "what matters most" (Yang et al. 2014) for those affected. Most importantly, the promise of mental health for all cannot be realized without addressing the complex social and structural determinants of mental illness whose solutions lie beyond the realm of individualized treatment whether from healers or psychiatrists.

## References

Ae-Ngibise, K., S. Cooper, E. Adiibokah, B. Akpalu, C. Lund, and V. Doku 2010 Whether you like it or not people with mental problems are going to go to them: A qualitative exploration into the widespread use of traditional and faith healers in the provision of mental health care in Ghana. International Review of Psychiatry 22 (6):558–567.

Aina, O. F. 2004 Mental illness and cultural issues in West African films: Implications for orthodox psychiatric practice. Medical Humanities 30 (1):23–26.

Akyeampong, E. 1996 Drink, Power, and Cultural Change: A Social History of Alcohol in Ghana, c. 1800 to Recent Times. Oxford: Heinemann.

Akyeampong, E., and P. Obeng 1995 Spirituality, gender, and power in Asante history. International Journal of African Historical Studies 28 (3):481–508.

Anas, A. A. 2009 Exposed: Inside Ghana's "mad house". The New Crusading Guide, 21 December. www.news.myjoyonline.com/news/200912/39569.asp.

Andersen, H. M. 2004 "Villagers": Differential treatment in a Ghanaian hospital. Social Science and Medicine 59 (10):2003–2012.

Appiah-Kubi, K. 1981 Man Cures, God Heals: Religion and Medical Practice Among the Akans of Ghana. New Jersey: Allanheld, Osmun and Co.

Ayim-Aboagye, D. 1993. The Function of Myth in Akan Healing Experience: A Psychological Inquiry into Two Traditional Akan Healing Communities. Uppsala: Acta Universitatis Upsaliensis.

Béhague, D., C. Tawiah, M. Rosato, T. Some, and J. Morrison 2009 Evidence-based policy-making: The implications of globally-applicable research for context-specific problem-solving in developing countries. Social Science and Medicine 69 (10):1539–1546.

Brodwin, P. 1996 Medicine and Morality in Haiti: The Contest for Healing Power. Cambridge: Cambridge University Press.

Campbell-Hall, V., I. Petersen, A. Bhana, S. Mjadu, V. Hosegood, A. J. Flisher, and MHaPP Research Programme Consortium. 2010 Collaboration between traditional practitioners and primary health care staff in South Africa: Developing a workable partnership for community mental health services. Transcultural Psychiatry 47 (4):610–628.

Dennis-Antwi, J. A., L. Culley, D. R. Hiles, and S. M. Dyson 2011 "I can die today, I can die tomorrow": Lay perceptions of sickle cell disease in Kumasi, Ghana at a point of transition. Ethnicity and Health 16 (4-5):465–481.

Feierman, S. 1985 Struggles for control: The social roots of health and healing in modern Africa. African Studies Review 28 (2/3):73–147.

———. 2000 Explanation and Uncertainty in the Medical World of Ghaambo. Bulletin of the History of Medicine 74 (2):317–344.

Field, M. J. 1955 Witchcraft as a primitive interpretation of mental disorder. Journal of Mental Science 101:826–833.

———. 1960. Search for Security: An Ethno-Psychiatric Study of Rural Ghana. London: Faber and Faber.

Fosu, G. B. 1981 Disease classification in rural Ghana: Framework and implications for health behaviour. Social Science and Medicine 15B:471–482.

Geschiere, P. 1997 The Modernity of Witchcraft: Politics and the Occult in Post-Colonial Africa. Charlottesville; London: University Press of Virginia.

Gilbert, M. 1989 Sources of power in Akuropon-Akuapem: Ambiguity in classification. *In* Creativity of Power: Cosmology and Creation in African Societies. W. Arens and I. Karp, eds. Pp. 59–90. Washington; London: Smithsonian Institution Press.

Graveling, E. 2010 "That is not religion, that is the gods": Ways of conceiving religious practices in rural Ghana. Culture and Religion 11 (1):31–50.

Gureje, O., V. O. Lasebikan, O. Ephraim-Oluwanuga, B. O. Olley, and L. Kola 2005 Community study of knowledge of and attitude to mental illness in Nigeria. British Journal of Psychiatry 186:436–441.

Halliburton, M. 2004 Finding a Fit: Psychiatric Pluralism in South India and its Implications for WHO Studies of Mental Disorder. Transcultural Psychiatry 41 (1):80–98.

Hampshire, K. R., and S. A. Owusu 2013 Grandfathers, Google, and dreams: Medical pluralism, globalization, and new healing encounters in Ghana. Medical Anthropology 32 (3):247–65.

Horton, R. 1967 African traditional thought and Western science. Africa 37 (1):50–71.

———. 2001 Ghana: Defining the African challenge. The Lancet 358 (9299):2141–9.

Human Rights Watch. 2012 Like a Death Sentence: Abuses against Persons with Mental Disabilities in Ghana.

Ingstad, B. 1995 *Mpho ya Modimo*—A gift from God: Perspectives on "attitudes" towards disabled persons. *In* Disabilty and Culture. B. Ingstad and S. R. Whyte, eds. Pp. 246–263. Berkeley: University of California Press.

Jain, S., and S. Jadhav 2009 Pills that swallow policy: Clinical ethnography of a community mental health program in northern India. Transcultural Psychiatry 46 (1):60–85.

Konadu, K. 2007 Indigenous Medicine and Knowledge in African Society. London: Routledge.

Lancet Global Mental Health Group 2007 Scale up services for mental disorders: A call for action. The Lancet 370 (9594):1241–1252.

Last, M. 1981 The importance of knowing about not knowing. Social Science & Medicine 15 (3):387–392.

Lewis, S., and J. Lieberman 2008 CATIE and CUtLASS: Can we handle the truth? British Journal of Psychiatry 192 (3):161–3.

McCall, J. C. 2003 Madness, money, and movies: Watching a Nigerian popular video with the guidance of a native doctor. Africa Today 49 (3):79–94.

McCaskie, T C. 1981 Anti-witchcraft cults in Asante: An essay in the social history of an African people. History in Africa 8:125–154.

———. 1995 State and Society in Pre-Colonial Asante. Cambridge: Cambridge University Press.

Meyer, B. 1999 Translating the Devil: Religion and Modernity among the Ewe in Ghana. Edinburgh: Edinburgh University Press.

———. 2003 Visions of blood, sex and money: Fantasy spaces in popular Ghanaian cinema. Visual Anthropology 16:15–41.

Minkus, H. K. 1980 The concept of spirit in Akwapim Akan philosophy. Africa 50 (2):182–192.

Morris, B. 2011 Medical herbalism in Malawi. Anthropology & Medicine 18 (2):245–255.

Mullings, L. 1984 Therapy, Ideology and Social Change: Mental Healing in Urban Ghana. Berkeley: University of California Press.

Offiong, D. A. 1999 Traditional healers in the Nigerian health care delivery system and the debate over integrating traditional and scientific medicine. Anthropological Quarterly 72 (3):118–130.

Orr, D. M. R. 2012 Patterns of persistence amidst medical pluralism: Pathways toward cure in the southern Peruvian Andes. Medical Anthropology 31 (6):514–530.

Patel, V., and G. Thornicroft 2009 Packages of care for mental, neurological, and substance use disorders in low- and middle-income countries. PLoS Med 6 (10):e1000160.

Peglidou, A. 2010 Therapeutic itineraries of "depressed" women in Greece: Power relationships and agency in therapeutic pluralism. Anthropology & Medicine 17 (1):41–57.

Pigg, S. L. 1996 The credible and the credulous: The question of "villagers' beliefs" in Nepal. Cultural Anthropology 11 (2):160–201.

Read, U. M. 2012 "I want the one that will heal me completely so it won't come back again": The limits of antipsychotic medication in rural Ghana. Transcultural Psychiatry 49 (3):1–23.

Romanucci-Ross, L. 1969 The hierarchy of resort in curative practices: The Admiralty Islands, Melanesia. Journal of Health and Social Behavior 10 (3):201–209.

*Read*

Strathern, M. 1988 The Gender of the Gift: Problems with Women and Problems with Society in Melanesia. Berkeley: University of California Press.

Stroeken, K. 2012 Health care decisions by Sukuma "peasant intellectuals": A case of radical empiricism? Anthropology & Medicine 19 (1):119–128.

Turner, V. W. 1967 The Forest of Symbols: Aspects of Ndembu Ritual. New York: Cornell University Press.

Ventevogel, P. 1996 Whiteman's Things: Training and De-training Healers in Ghana. Amsterdam: Het Spinhuis.

Whyte, S. R. 1992 Pharmaceuticals as folk medicine: Transformations in the social relations of health care in Uganda. Culture, Medicine and Psychiatry 16:163–186.

———. 2012 Chronicity and control: Framing "noncommunicable diseases" in Africa. Anthropology & Medicine 19 (1):63–74.

Yang, L. H., F. Chen, K. J. Sia, J. Lam, K. Lam, H. Ngo, S. Lee, A. Kleinman, and B. Good 2014 "What matters most:" A cultural mechanism moderating structural vulnerability and moral experience of mental illness stigma. Social Science & Medicine 103 (0):84–93.

# Chapter 9

## The Person in Between: Discourses on Madness, Money and Magic in Malawi

*Arne S. Steinforth*

**Introduction**

When I first started conducting research on the local construction of mental disorder in Southern Malawi in 2004, I was prepared to find that a significant part of local discourses on the topic would revolve around, in the broadest sense of the word, religious notions. My subsequent results not only corroborated this initial hypothesis but significantly surpassed my expectations. For clinical psychiatrists, the multitude of ideas surrounding mental disorder constitutes a considerable challenge.

In order to address the different ways in which people with mental health problems in settings like Malawi conceive of their situation, numerous studies have, from a clinical perspective, classified clients according to a three-tiered model of personhood—differentiating a Traditional from a Modern (also Westernized or Therapeutic) and, in between the two, a Transitional (or Mixed) Type (cf., e.g., Boroffka 2006; Peltzer 1987). As modifications of such heuristic models, more psychological analytic approaches classify the different configurations of the self as egocentric, sociocentric, ecocentric and cosmocentric (see Kirmayer 2007), thereby offering a more comprehensive outlook on the relatedness between a given concept of the person, its dominant values and locus of agency and the most suitable healing system within it.

All these classificatory models give telling evidence not only of the simultaneous coexistence of different concepts of the person in a given society but also of the considerable relevance of such concepts within the therapeutic process. All of them can further be assumed to imply that prevalent concepts of personhood are connected to larger processes of social transformation, and that the influence of globalized European ideas entails a spread of more individualist, Westernized notions of the person in these postcolonial settings.

It is this dynamic dimension of specific concepts of the person that this article means to investigate. The seemingly long-winded question it explores may be summarized as follows: if the specific concept of the person is indeed essential for the efficiency of psychotherapeutic methods applied in cases of mental health disorder, and if postcolonial socio-political developments inevitably bring about the proliferation of more European ideas and values into societies, e.g., in sub-Saharan Africa, then is it safe to assume that this ongoing change will lead to a gradual transformation of "non-modern," non-individualistic notions of the person, thus making future mental health clients in these settings more readily receptive to European notions of mental health and, hence, to its well-established psychotherapeutic armamentarium? Or, to pose the question in more general terms: can the postcolonial person—who, in the past, has been labeled as unsuitable for European psychotherapy due to an assumed fundamental otherness (cf. Carothers 1954; Gilman 1985; Mahone 2007; McCulloch 1995; Stubbe 2008)—be expected to become so deeply Europeanized by the universalizing effects of globalization that existing differences in mental care needs will, finally, be leveled out?

Obviously, this is a broad and complex question to engage with. With all due caution, I mean to offer a tentative answer by focusing on the present-day situation in a given African setting. Focusing on recent transformations in local discourses on mental health, this paper seeks to demonstrate the necessity to distinguish between two levels of analysis, namely that of the concept of the person on the one hand—and, underneath it, that of alternative systems of values. In so doing, it concludes that the relevance of religion as a vast body of ideas through which mental disorder may be addressed has proven remarkably resilient to global processes of modernization.[1]

---

[1] The empirical data this article draws upon was collected during more than two years of field research, conducted in different phases between 2004 and 2010. For facilitating the realization of research, I am indebted to the German Academic Exchange Service (DAAD) as well as Helene Basu and the Cluster of Excellence "Religion and Politics" at WWU Münster.

## Cosmologies of Mental Disorder

Throughout long periods of field research in different rural and urban settings in Southern Malawi, my local counterparts attributed cases of mental disorder largely to secret ritual machinations of other persons or the actions of non-human spirit entities. For the sake of analysis, I found it instrumental to classify local aetiological models into three main categories—i.e., into notions of structural, spiritual and personal causation of mental disorder (Steinforth 2009).[2]

Structural causation—as the first and least prevalent of the three—represents the closest equivalent to, e.g., European notions of mental disorder, which manifests itself due to personal life experiences, sudden neurological imbalances or genetic predisposition. It implies that neither person nor spirit entity are seen as being directly or intentionally involved in causing the given condition—thereby representing a case frequently verbalized (in Chichewa, the national language of Malawi alongside English) by expressions such as *zimachitika* or "things just happen." In most instances when such an explanation was drawn upon, the specific cases were related to drug abuse (mostly of *chamba*, or Indian hemp), accidents (especially those related to damage sustained to the head) and inheritance (in the sense of a faulty mental condition being passed on from generation to generation along the line of blood).

Secondly, spiritual causation comprises a broad range of cases in which non-human spirit entities of different kinds are identified as the immediate reason for mental disorder. Such incidents include spiritual intervention in the shape of, e.g., an ancestor spirit (*mzimu wa makolo*) causing mental disorder to a sometimes purposefully, sometimes randomly selected descendant in order to substantiate a particular claim (such as for the group to hold a second funeral ritual, for some descendants to resume

---

[2] The following section summarizes some results published previously in the referenced monograph (Steinforth 2009). For the sake of this paper, I have subjected my own analysis to a partial re-examination, therefore renaming the category previously addressed "magic manipulation" as "personal causation." In so doing, I mean to avoid the "heavy ideological baggage" (Ellis and Ter Haar 2013) connected to the concept of magic and other similarly elusive categories. Notwithstanding these reservations, the short and maybe all too lurid catchword "magic" is still allowed to feature in the title of this paper.

giving regular libations or for a given person to take up work as a *sing'anga* healer). Likewise, however, the attacks of malevolent spirit entities also fall under this category. In local terms, this may include the malicious and strictly destructive actions of the non-human and therefore non-social *ziwanda* spirits from the bush, or, from a more strongly Muslim or Christian perspective, this may be addressed as satanic forces (i.e., demons or *majini* spirits) who also endeavor to inflict pain and suffering on the living with no moral justification whatsoever. And lastly, the will of God (or, in more rarely reported Muslim accounts, Allah) may also be identified as the ultimate rationale for the occurrence of mental disorder—in terms of an either generalized or specific form of divine punishment. In some cases, Christian (and frequently Pentecostal) counterparts described the non-normative behavior of a person as the reason for his or her particular vulnerability to demonic aggression. After all, close spiritual proximity to Jesus Christ as the "ultimate healer" (Schoffeleers 1994) is regarded as the quintessential source of protection against all kinds of satanic influence, and those who stray from the path of the godly inevitably become targets of demonic attacks. In some cases, however, it was also argued that the will of God (*chifuniro cha Mulungu*, sometimes also phrased as *mphatso ya Mulungu*, therefore a "gift from God") may cause mental disorder to any person, indiscriminate of their actions, in order to remind the living of the supreme divine power and urge them towards humility and normative behavior.

Thirdly, personal causation suggests that other living persons are identified as willfully causing mental disorder in another person by the use of secret rituals which, in anthropological literature, have usually been described in terms of "magic," "sorcery" or "witchcraft." As the most prominent of these concepts, *ufiti* (witchcraft) is defined as the evil doings of persons who, due to their contamination with a mysterious *ufiti* substance, are working tirelessly to hurt, harm or kill their fellow human beings at night by means of secret techniques—and who are motivated by jealousy, malice and hatred. Mental disorder is frequently rumored to be the outcome of *ufiti* activities because it incapacitates a whole family by not only eliminating the workforce of one of its members but by further necessitating family care. *Kutsilika* rituals, on the other hand (meaning "protection" and also addressed as *matsenga*, or "sorcery"), are performed quite openly—especially for the purpose of protecting property—and are usually part of the expertise provided by Malawian healers *(a-*

*sing'anga*). These kinds of rituals feature prominently in mental health narratives—and whenever this is the case, they usually assume that the person suffering from mental disorder must have laid hands on property that was ritually protected against burglary.

Finally, as a third form of personal causation that is of particular importance to the argument of this paper, certain secret rituals are known to be used for the sake of attaining personal power or wealth (Chilivumbo 1976; Lwanda 2005; Marwick 1965; Peltzer 1987). According to this notion locally addressed as *kukhwima* (and translated as "to fortify oneself"), an aspiring person addresses a ritual expert (usually a *sing'anga* healer) and expresses the personal goal he or she hopes to achieve. The expert then provides the customer with the necessary secret instructions (*zizimba*) which invariably include the breach of central social norms such as the customer committing incest by having sex with a close relative (usually a sister or mother), or by ritually sacrificing a family member's mental capacities and well-being.

This is where mental disorder becomes a prominent issue featuring in *kukhwima* narratives in two distinct ways. Firstly, any ambitious person who, after having received ritual instructions from an expert, fails to perform the demanded actions in minute detail—either due to compunction, carelessness or other reasons—will be inevitably struck with mental disorder.[3] The second line of narrative relies on local ideas that the users of *kukhwima* rituals are required to "steal" the personal spirit (*mzimu wa umunthu*, see below) of a family member in order to achieve the desired goal, thus sacrificing the victim's mental health and rendering him or her in a state of severe mental disorder.

The high prevalence of ideas of personal or spiritual causation for mental disorder in Malawi is supported by studies from psychiatrists. By 1995, a study on social psychiatry assessed that the majority of clients admitted to Zomba Mental Hospital (up to now the country's only governmental psychiatric institution) described their own condition with reference to, as the authors phrase it, "traditional" concepts (MacLachlan, Nyirenda, and

---

[3] Very pragmatically, some accounts mention that the unwillingness of, e.g., a woman to comply with her brother's ritual obligation of having sexual intercourse with her is a known reason for clients finding themselves unable to carry out *zizimba* instructions.

Nyando 1995)—which encompass both the categories of spiritual and personal causation described above. More recently, clinical psychiatrists I interviewed have estimated that about 60 percent of those persons admitted to Zomba Mental Hospital attribute their own suffering to reasons that would qualify as personal causation—with another large percentage of clients relating their condition to spiritual reasons. One Malawian psychiatrist phrased his perspective on the social specificity of motifs that are applied in mental disorder as follows:

> Most delusions in Malawi follow religious symbols. When I was working in Australia, typical delusions were attacking UFOs, or the TV controlling your mind. Back here in Malawi, there is none of that, but lots on witchcraft, spirit possession and the like. [Stewart Chipendo, personal communication]

Not surprisingly, the overall approach of Malawian psychiatrists tends to differ significantly from that of the general population, including their clients who maintain a strong association of mental disorder with spiritual or personal lines of causation.[4] In particular, the association of mental disorder with secret *kukhwima* practices was extremely prevalent during the time of my research, and many accounts described this as a very recent occurrence.

This same perceived change in the nature of mental disorder is not only prevalent among the poorly educated, rural majority of the population. In this very same vein, a successful Malawian businesswoman in the capital of Lilongwe told me that she had recently stopped giving money to anyone begging on the streets because "most of them did it to themselves, or someone in their own family did it to them. They want to become rich fast, and so they do evil things. They themselves are the ones to blame" (Gladys Chamangwana, personal communication).

Strikingly, while the notion of *kukhwima* as explicated above is not mentioned in earlier studies on mental health in Malawi (Peltzer 1987), by 2004 it had become so widespread that, indeed, its sudden prevalence was commented upon by staff members of Zomba Mental Hospital. When asked, one Malawian psychiatrist exclaimed: "Do I hear a lot about *ku-*

---

[4] As the abovementioned psychiatrist told me, "If you ask me, witchcraft is a delusion. But that's just my opinion" (Stewart Chipendo, personal communication).

*khwima*? It is like an epidemic in Zomba Mental Hospital!" (Stewart Chipendo, personal communication).

So, if a cosmological concept such as *kukhwima* has such a high degree of prominence within mental health discourse by 2004 while being absent from studies conducted in the late 1980s, does this indicate a noticeable transformation of the local conceptualization of mental disorder? And, if so, how can this transformation be connected to larger social processes in Malawi?

**Market Economy and the Madness of Success**

According to emic Malawian discourse, the occurrence of secret *kukhwima* rituals is intrinsically related to postcolonial history. When Malawi gained its national independence in 1964, British colonialism was replaced by a similarly oppressive and dictatorial regime led by the self-appointed Life President Hastings Kamuzu Banda. Banda's government was marked by an explicit attempt to minimize external influence on the mostly rural farming communities of the country. International newspapers were banned, TV and radio programs tightly supervised and heavily censored and immigrant groups within the country—such as the considerable Indian trading community—were allowed to settle only in designated areas of the country so as not to expose the average Malawian to non-Malawian ideas and practices. In so doing, Banda's regime managed to maintain a sharp distinction between a small, well-educated, globally informed and economically prosperous elite and the overwhelming majority of the population, who were encouraged to value their small-scale farming, extended family structure and rich village life.

This rigid system, in which the place of any given person was virtually predefined by birth, changed dramatically in 1994 when the introduction of multiparty democracy led to the presidency of Bakili Muluzi. As a successful businessman, Muluzi set into motion a far-reaching liberalization of the national economy that not only paved the way for previously unprecedented amounts of development aid and foreign investment pouring into Malawi but also sparked the idea that, through private entrepreneurship and personal ambition, economic success was finally within reach of every part of the population. This new age of an apparently unlimited social upward mobility (sometimes mockingly addressed as the

"Malawian Dream") was further nurtured through the growing availability of South African, European, North American and other mass media in the form of international newspapers, TV shows and the Internet. Through these channels of information, new images of globalized ideas of what everybody's life should be like made their impact felt even on the grassroots level.

The political changes of 1994 mark the beginning of a new—and, to use a recent buzzword, neoliberal—economic system that, according to public discourse, is in turn closely linked with a rising occurrence of *kukhwima* practices. My Malawian counterparts invariably agreed that, in the past, knowledge about this form of secret rituals used to be a privilege of office-holders (such as village headmen and elders); they harbored, employed and controlled access to that ritual knowledge as a means to insure their own elevated social rank and, by extension, to uphold social order as a whole. In their role as living representations and ritual "owners of the land" (*eni dziko*), local chiefs (*mafumu*) were charged with the responsibility of safeguarding the well-being of the community—an obligation that set them apart from the more generally accepted confines of morality and normative behavior (Kaspin 1990; Probst 2005; Wishlade 1961). Now, it appears that postcolonial developments have led to a mainstreaming of the idea of rapid, spiritually induced personal success that is disconnected from public office.

Such a separation of personal achievement from the social office, argues Jean La Fontaine (1985), is a clear indicator for the introduction of individualist ideas into society. From this vantage point, it therefore becomes feasible to think of *kukhwima* (and the changed public perspective on mental disorder closely related to it) as an expression of larger social transformations in postcolonial and post-dictatorial Malawi which challenge and transform preexisting notions of the relationship between the person and society as a whole. It further appears evident that the social deregulation of *kukhwima* as an alleged tool for ritually precipitating personal success is indeed linked to processes of monetization and individualization related to the realities of a Western notion of modernity, thus qualifying as an expression of an "occult economy" (Comaroff and Comaroff 1999). The question still remains, however, whether the evidently increasing influence of individualist ideas within Malawian society can be expected to lead to a fundamental reformulation of local concepts of the person that will make average Malawians more suitable clients to Western psychotherapy.

**Persons in Transition?**

In Malawi, sets of explicitly validated social values and norms of behavior feature strongly in local institutions such as initiatory teachings, behavioral guidelines and proverbs. Taken together, they form a fairly consistent picture of how Malawian society defines socially moral behavior. Condensing these notions makes it feasible, as I argue, to deduce an ideal model of the person that is associated with morality and life in the rural communities which orbits around key values such as interdependence, reliability, cooperation, modesty, conformity, low levels of social stratification and strongly collectivist orientations within the community. According to Brian Morris (1994), the great importance of collectivist values in Malawi and many other African societies effectively discourages open self-assertion and self-aggrandizement, leading to what Robert LeVine (1982) calls a "norm of humility."

In European societies, it is somewhat of a stereotype for especially elderly people to lament the loss of morality in present times, and to refer to the past in terms of a more wholesome, more just, or more desirable time when the social vices of the present day were as yet unknown. The same holds true for a large percentage of my Malawian counterparts who deplore that, nowadays, more and more of their fellow countrypeople think only of their own material gain—rather than considering the integrity of their families and adhering to the way of life of their forefathers. This criticism revolves around very clear ideas of ethical, normative social behavior that demarcates explicit boundaries between the personal needs, wishes and ambitions of the individual and the social demands, expectations and roles of the community. Accordingly, the abovementioned set of values represented in social institutions is complemented by another model that, according to local discourse, is related to more recent ideas and foreign influence. This alternative set of values is based on criteria such as autonomy, flexibility, competition, achievement, uniqueness and social hierarchy as defined by economic success, thus showing a much more directly individualist outlook on the person. In themselves, these values are associated with urban lifestyle, which goes along with more strongly materialist interests including the public display of wealth and symbols of a Western, globalized modernity.

In total, the conflict expressed in this kind of social discourse clusters around two distinct and ideal typical sets of social values that I will use here as a heuristic tool for better understanding the local dynamics of social transformation: the Home Village Ideal and the Big City Ideal. In this binary constellation, the Home Village Ideal essentially features as the model of a moral life, identified with rural lifestyle, agricultural production and a strong commitment to family and community; the Big City Ideal, on the other hand, represents the model of a pleasant life associated with urban lifestyle, wage labor and a relative independence from family and community obligations. In this dynamic picture of a slow process of disintegration of long-held local norms, the Malawian person seems stuck between these two supposedly "traditional" versus "modern" sets of values. This constitutes what, from my perspective, can be considered a conflict between different systems of values between which the person is located.

It is at this point that we return to the initial question of how this apparent social transformation reflects on the concept of the person. Whenever I asked my Malawian counterparts about their understanding of the person (or *munthu*), their answer usually indicated a tripartite concept of components (La Fontaine 1985; Morris 1994:123–147; Tempels 1959 [1945]). Firstly, the human body (*thupi*) is described as the material vessel that is subject to growth, change and decay. Secondly, this body is animated by a "divine spirit" (*mzimu wa umulungu*), the spark of life or vital force. This spirit is described as given by God, as received during conception, as unchanging during lifetime and as returning to the Creator upon the person's death (cf. Chigona 2002; Steinforth 2009). As the last component, the so-called earthly or "human spirit" (*mzimu wa umunthu*) is regarded as the faculty that controls a person's decision-making processes and voluntary actions. It changes throughout one's lifetime, grows by personal experience and is identical with the part of a person's metaphysical existence that transforms into an ancestral spirit (*mzimu wa makolo*) after death.

While this three-part model seems to be a prominent reference point in local discourse, the local understanding of the human person also relates to certain qualities or competences that are defined as belonging to a normal human being. The criteria that therefore further qualify a person include factors such as (1) economic productivity and (2) procreativity (i.e., capacity to reproduce), but also (3) social interaction and responsibility within the family and community and (4) compliance with basic cultural norms including respect towards elders as well as the maintenance of functioning relationships with the cosmological sphere—either conceived of as ancestor spirits (*mizimu ya makolo*) or as God in Christian or Muslim terms.

There is certainly a lot more to be said on the concept of the person. For the sake of this paper, it may suffice to assert that, in Malawi as in many other settings worldwide, social relations as well as cosmological ones play a constitutive part in what marks full human competence and, therefore, personhood. This specific conception of the person is based on an idea of social and cosmological connectedness that defines the person in strongly relational, socio-cosmological terms (cf. Kirmayer 2007). Throughout my research, there was no indication that this outlook on the person's place within society and cosmos is undergoing any fundamental, rapid and imminent change. Rather, people in Malawi have a tendency to complain about the rise of individualistic values within society while holding on to the concept of the person defined by social and cosmological relatedness. What, therefore, are the implications if, as Laurence Kirmayer (2007) and others have suggested, the goals of psychotherapeutic treatment are tied to the culturally specific concept of the person (Corin 1998)? What does it mean for the Malawian practice of psychotherapy if most of its methods are developed in European and North American contexts and based on an individualistic conception of the person?

To answer this question, I need to add another dimension to the problem. From the perspective of the anthropology of religion or medical anthropology, one of the most well-reported transformations in the Malawian landscape of healing that took place in the last two decades has indeed been the remarkable rise of Pentecostal churches (Englund 2007; Fiedler 1999; Strohbehn 2005; van Dijk 2002). Most adherents of Pentecostal churches I have interviewed insist that their miraculous powers of healing are indeed the main motive for conversion—not only in Malawi but on a global scale. Yet, despite their tapping into globalized discourses of religion by using symbolisms of North American and West African televangelism in their performances, the healing ministry of these churches that represents a key feature to their proliferation is not based on an individualistic model of the person. Rather, it offers collective ritual within which the congregation takes on the role of an extended family, and where the direct incorporation of the Holy Spirit acts as the quintessential key to personal healing (Gunther Brown 2011; Kalu 2008). It follows that from a local perspective, their form of worship and healing— even if incorporating some individualist ideas—maintains the overall concept of the person that strongly emphasizes the socio-cosmological relatedness of the person. In spite of the remarkable social changes that people in Malawi perceive and which they associate with the occurrence of mental disorder, the socio-cosmological orientation of the person remains intact. Therefore, the great impact of allegedly new, individualist notions in emic Malawian discourse is not directed at the concept of the person itself, but at the level of social values on which the former is grounded. Ultimately, the tension between opposing sets of values should then not be understood as an irreversible break between one model and the other, but rather as a pluralization of the landscape of social values that makes it possible for the person to access alternative frames of reference when locating themselves within society.

**Conclusion**

In my opinion, my Malawian data indicates that, within this given social setting, the occurrence of mental disorder is strongly associated with recent processes of social transformation and with a perceived loss of social cohesion that comes with it. This, however, does not diminish the fact that both idealized ends of this process are locally framed in socio-cosmological terms. If the changes within Malawian society that I have looked at (and that are locally perceived as being the most noteworthy) may indeed be addressed as the introduction of a European–North American concept of the individual, then this idea is itself transformed to fit into a profoundly socio-cosmological concept of personhood and society. The social transformation that is indicated by the sudden rise of *kukhwima* as a local idiom for both personal gain and suffering can, at least so far, not be identified as a unilinear development towards a structurally new, Westernized idea. Rather, it appears to represent a pluralization of social values that, while producing strong social tension and personal conflict, remains deeply rooted in relational, non-individualist notions of the person.

It has already been established that different models of locating the person within society may well coexist and be referred to alternatively (Corin 1998; Kirmayer 2007:246). After all, claims at establishing a clear-cut binary division between African collectivism and European individualism have been cautioned by Morris (1994) and many others (e.g., Heinz 2006; Kirmayer 2007) who identify this as a grave oversimplification of affairs. All societies have their own mechanisms of negotiating the goals of the person against those of society as a whole. But while the dichotomy between collectivist and individualist orientations of the person may not hold true on the analytical level, it may indeed hold some powerful leverage on the level of emic discourse.

From this vantage point, it becomes all the more apparent why institutions such as Zomba Mental Hospital in Malawi find it hard to be locally accepted as a viable therapeutic option for addressing mental disorder. Persons admitted to its wards—many of whom, as I have argued, are aware of their mental disorder but think of their condition in terms of spirits, witchcraft or *kukhwima* rituals—consider themselves in the wrong place because their personal therapeutic needs cannot be met. On the basis of my argument that a fundamental transformation in the general understanding of the person, society and mental disorder does not appear to be forthcoming anytime soon in Malawi, it becomes all the more elementary for changes to be introduced on the side of therapeutic institutions in order to better accommodate the needs of the contemporary setup of both Malawian society and the person.

This conclusion may hardly be news to some, yet it appears to be a point that needs to be remade. The same conceptual ground has already been broken on the African continent more than 50 years ago. Through the realization of the Aro village system in Nigeria in the 1950s, Adeoye Lambo and his collaborators—including outstanding psychiatric personalities such as Alexander Leighton, Raymond Prince or German psychiatrist Alexander Boroffka—have addressed this same issue (Adewunmi 2002; Asuni 1967; Ayonrinde, Gureje, and Lawal 2004; Boroffka 2006; Lambo 1961; Leighton et al. 1963; Sadowsky 1999). Accordingly, the most immediate structural reforms they implemented in this project included not only a system of family or community care but also the direct therapeutic involvement of local, non-Western-trained practitioners, thereby reflecting the same social and cosmological relatedness of the person that is evident in my Malawian case.

The observations I have elaborated on do not constitute a specifically African phenomenon, nor are they limited to postcolonial societies or intrinsically connected to migrant populations. Rather, the European–North American concept of the person as an individual, autonomous and self-reliant entity and, at the same time, as the building block of an allegedly modern and therefore secular society should itself be subjected to further and thorough scrutiny.

**References**

Adewunmi, A. 2002 Community Psychiatry in Nigeria. The Psychiatrist 26:394–395.

Asuni, T. 1967 Aro Hospital in Perspective. American Journal of Psychiatry 124(6):763–770.

Ayonrinde, O., O. Gureje, and R. Lawal 2004 Psychiatric Research in Nigeria: Bridging Tradition and Modernisation. The British Journal of Psychiatry 184:536–538.

Boroffka, A. 2006 Psychiatry in Nigeria (a Partly Annotated Bibliography) with an Introductory Chapter on "the History of Psychiatry in Nigeria". Kiel: Brunswicker Universitäts-Buchhandlung.

Carothers, J. C. 1954 The Psychology of Mau Mau: Colony and Protectorate of Kenya. Nairobi: Government Press.

Chigona, G. 2002 Umunthu Theology: Path of Integral Human Liberation Rooted in Jesus of Nazareth. Balaka: Montford Media.

Chilivumbo, A. B. 1976 Social Basis of Illness: A Search for Therapeutic Meaning. *In* Medical Anthropology. F. X. Grollig and H. B. Haley, eds. Pp. 67–79. Den Haag: Mouton Publisher.

Comaroff, J., and J. L. Comaroff. 1999 Occult Economies and the Violence of Abstraction: Notes from the South African Postcolony. American Ethnologist 26(2):279–303.

Corin, E. 1998. Refiguring the Person: The Dynamics of Affects and Symbols in an African Spirit Possession Cult. *In* Bodies and Persons:

Comparative Perspectives from Africa and Melanesia. M. Lambek and A. Strathern, eds. Pp. 80–102. New York: Cambridge University Press.

Ellis, S., and G. Ter Haar. 2013 Spirits in Politics: Some Theoretical Reflections. *In* Spirits in Politics: Uncertainties of Power and Healing in African Societies. B. Meier and A. S. Steinforth, eds. Pp. 37–48. Frankfurt: Campus.

Englund, H. 2007 Pentecostalism beyond Belief: Trust and Democracy in a Malawian Township. Africa 77(4):477–499.

Fiedler, K. 1999 Charismatic and Pentecostal Movements in Malawi in Cultural Perspective. Religion in Malawi 9:27–38.

Gilman, S. 1985 Difference and Pathology: Stereotypes of Sexuality, Race, and Madness. Ithaca, NY: Cornell University Press.

Gunther Brown, C. 2011 Global Pentecostal and Charismatic Healing. New York: Oxford University Press.

Heinz, A. 2006 Die Konzeption des ‚Selbst' im kulturellen Vergleich. *In* Transkulturelle Psychiatrie–Interkulturelle Psychotherapie: Interdisziplinäre Theorie und Praxis. E. Wohlfart and M. Zaumseil, eds. Pp. 377–390. Heidelberg: Springer.

Kalu, O. 2008 African Pentecostalism: An Introduction. Oxford: Oxford University Press.

Kaspin, D. 1990 Elephants and Ancestors: The Legacy of Kingship in Rural Malawi. Chicago: University of Chicago Press.

Kirmayer, L. J. 2007 Psychotherapy and the Cultural Concept of the Person. Transcultural Psychiatry 44:232–257.

La Fontaine, J. S. 1985 Person and Individual: Some Anthropological Reflections. *In* The Category of the Person: Anthropology, Philosophy, History. M. Carrithers, S. Collins, and S. Lukes, eds. Pp. 123–140. Cambridge: Cambridge University Press.

Lambo, T. A. 1961 A Form of Social Psychiatry in Africa. World Mental Health 13(4):190–203.

Leighton, A. H., T. A. Lambo, C. C. Hughes, D. C. Leighton, J. M. Murphy, and D. B. Macklin 1963 Psychiatric Disorder among the Yoruba: A Report from the Cornell-Aro Mental Health Research Project in the Western Region, Nigeria. Ithaca, NY: Cornell University Press.

LeVine, R. A. 1982 The Self and Its Development in an African Society. *In* Psychosocial Theories of the Self. B. Lee, ed. Pp. 43–65. New York: Plenum Press.

Lwanda, J. L. C. 2005. Politics, Culture and Medicine in Malawi. Zomba: Kachere Series.

MacLachlan, M., T. Nyirenda, and C. Nyando 1995 Attributions for Admission to Zomba Mental Hospital: Implications for the Development of Mental Health Services in Malawi. International Journal of Social Psychiatry 41(2):79–87.

Mahone, S. 2007 East African Psychiatry and the Practical Problems of Empire. *In* Psychiatry and Empire. S. Mahone and M. Vaughan, eds. Pp. 41–66. Basingstoke: Palgrave Macmillan.

Marwick, M. G. 1965 Sorcery in Its Social Setting: A Study of the North Rhodesian Chewa. Manchester: Manchester University Press.

McCulloch, J. 1995 Colonial Psychiatry and 'the African Mind'. Cambridge: Cambridge University Press.

Morris, B. 1994 Anthropology of the Self: The Individual in Cultural Perspective. London: Pluto Press.

Peltzer, K. 1987 Some Contributions of Traditional Healing Practices towards Psychosocial Health Care in Malawi. Eschborn: Fachbuchhandlung für Psychologie.

Probst, P. 2005 Kalumbas Fest: Lokalität, Geschichte und rituelle Praxis in Malawi. Münster: LIT-Verlag.

Sadowsky, J. H. 1999 Imperial Bedlam: Institutions of Madness in Colonial Southwest Nigeria. Berkeley: University of California Press.

Schoffeleers, M. 1994 Christ in African Folk Theology: The Nganga Paradigm. *In* Religion in Africa: Experience & Expression. T. D. Blakely, W. E. A. van Beek, and D. L. Thomson, eds. Pp. 73–88. London: James Currey.

Steinforth, A. S. 2009 Troubled Minds: On the Cultural Construction of Mental Disorder and Normality in Southern Malawi. Frankfurt: Peter Lang.

Strohbehn, U. 2005 Pentecostalism in Malawi: A History of the Apostolic Faith Mission 1931–1994. Zomba: Kachere Series.

Stubbe, H. 2008 Sigmund Freuds „Totem und Tabu" in Mosambik: Eine Psychologie-Historische Studie. Göttingen: V&R unipress.

Tempels, P. 1959 [1945] Bantu Philosophy. Paris: Présence Africaine.

van Dijk, R. 2002 Modernity's Limits: Pentecostalism and the Moral Rejection of Alcohol in Malawi. *In* Alcohol in Africa: Mixing Business, Pleasure and Politics. D. F. Bryceson, eds. Pp. 249–264. Portsmouth: Heinemann.

Wishlade, R. L. 1961 Chiefship and Politics in the Mlanje District of Southern Nyasaland. Africa. Journal of the International African Institute 31(1):36–45.

# Chapter 10

## The Experience of Healing and the Healing of Experience in the Pentecostal Movement

*Simon Dein*

### Introduction

In this chapter I examine the role of bodily experience in Pentecostal healing and more specifically the ways in which some Pentecostal groups have moved away from medical confirmation of the success of healing to criteria based upon bodily experiences. I begin by arguing for the centrality of healing in the Pentecostal movement before examining attitudes towards biomedicine and conceptualizations of sickness and healing in more detail. I then examine anthropological work in this area.

### Pentecostalism

As a definitive religious group, it has been estimated that Pentecostals number over 570 million adherents (Barrett and Johnson 2004), making it the largest non-Catholic group of Christians in the world, accounting for one in every four Christians (Dobbins 2000). It is estimated that Pentecostalism is the fastest growing denomination in Christianity—Cox (2011) refers to the phenomenon as a "New Reformation." Pentecostal and Charismatic Christianity is a global phenomenon that comprises a quarter of the world's two billion Christians and is growing rapidly (Gunther Brown 2011). According to the Pew Forum on Religion and Public Life (2006), Pentecostalism has grown according to researchers from 72 million in 1960 to 525 million in 2000 with the majority of growth occurring in non-Western countries in the Caribbean, South America and Africa (Barker 2005). In the West, the movement is strong in the black churches and the American and Australian "mega-churches" such as Hillsong Church and comprises a number of different churches which all similarly emphasize a belief in the physical manifestations of the Holy Spirit—particularly speaking in tongues. The movement has been inspired by the Festival of Pentecost marking the coming of the Holy Spirit to the Apostles 50 days after Easter where Jesus' disciples spoke in many languages as described in the Book of Acts: all of them were filled with the Holy Spirit and began to speak in other tongues as the Spirit enabled them (Acts 2:4).

I shall briefly outline the history of the Pentecostal movement. From the mid–19th century, a strand of the Holiness movement emerged which asserted that a second conversion experience was possible—adult baptism—in which the convert would be cleansed from sin. This, together with millennialism and a literal approach to scripture which promised spiritual gifts to believers, led to an increased interest in divine healing and other manifestations of the Holy Spirit. In 1906 there was a sudden manifestation of spiritual activity in Los Angeles in the Azusa Street Mission led by Charles Fox Parham, which has generally been regarded by historians as the birth of the Pentecostal movement. During the Azusa Street meetings, according to witnesses who wrote about them, blind, paralyzed or other sick people would reputedly be healed. A second form of Pentecostalism arose in the 1960s after many non-Pentecostals became aware of Pentecostalism through an earlier Pentecostal revival organized by faith-healing evangelists (notably Oral Roberts). The movement has been closely aligned with charismatic individuals and the style of worship is emotional with music, clapping chorusing and dynamic preaching. Dobbins (2000) remarks that there are three distinct groups included under the term "Pentecostal": classical Pentecostals (denominations formed in the early 20th century), Charismatics (mainline Protestants who endorse the Pentecostal experience) and Independents (independent churches unaffiliated with any parent organization).

Pentecostals hold traditional evangelical beliefs such as the existence of a personal God, the divinity of Jesus Christ, the divine inspiration of scripture and the sinful nature (i.e., predisposition to do wrong) of humans, who are in need of salvation through belief in the death and resurrection of Christ (Thiessen 1979). What differentiates Pentecostals from other evangelical Christians are doctrines focusing on the Holy Spirit and an emphasis on ecstatic experience—adherents believe that faith must be powerfully experiential, and not something found merely through ritual or thinking. Pentecostalism is "spirit driven" and adherents maintain that through a strong commitment to faith the Holy Spirit will become mani-

*Experience of Healing, Healing of Experience*

fest in them. In addition to the spiritual gifts including speaking in tongues, faith healing, prophecy and exorcism, many Pentecostals maintain that God rewards them materially and this manifests in the prosperity gospel. There is no universal stance on doctrine or polity among adherents, although in the US Pentecostals are generally conservative Evangelicals. Pentecostalism is theologically and historically close to the Charismatic movement as it significantly influenced that movement, and sometimes the terms Pentecostal and Charismatic are used interchangeably.

While the manifestation of spiritual gifts is central to the Pentecostal movement, we lack data on how commonly these spiritual gifts occur. Poloma (1989) surveyed members (N 1,275) of one large Pentecostal denomination (Assemblies of God) and found that 91 percent reported experiencing a "definite answer" to prayer requests, 67 percent had spoken in tongues, 62 percent believed they had experienced a miraculous healing within the past year, 50 percent heard God speak to them in a dream or vision and 30 percent experienced giving a prophecy. Thus it appears they are quite prevalent.

**Explanatory Models of Illness and Help Seeking**

Illness in the New Testament was generally attributed to God, the devil or demons, to sin or to natural causes. It ultimately derives from the fall and final healing is not possible until Christ returns. As Belcher and Hall (2001) note, 1 Corinthians 1:4–8 is an important scripture for many Pentecostals. The passage shows that the reason God provides spiritual gifts, such as healing, is to build up and maintain Christians until they "arrive" in his Parousia, which occurs at the end of time (Ruthven 1997). Healing represents an eschatological struggle which is temporary here on earth, and a fuller life is only possible at the Parousia or after death.

Sickness is often understood to be the result of demonic activity. These demons are seen as servants of Satan but not usually Satan himself. Although they are spiritual in nature they can operate through material bodies and are like the Holy Spirit, which can also possess a body and cause behaviors like speaking in tongues. Behaviors caused by spiritual entities indicate the presence of those entities; just as speaking in tongues indicates the presence of the Holy Spirit in the speaker, so too disturbed behaviors are indicators of the demonic presence. The type of mental illness which manifests itself is dependent on which spirit entity possesses an individual.

Hammond and Hammond (2010) list four pages of names for groupings of demons, including spirits of bitterness, rebellion, strife, control, nervousness and paranoia. Early childhood experiences can open "ports of entry" for demons leading to possession, including particularly adoption, parental consideration of abortion and childhood trauma. One's own experiences of physical sickness and death can "invite" demons to enter. Furthermore, experiences with the occult or curses can render a person susceptible to demonic influence.

There is recent research suggesting that cultural and ethnic groups conceptualize mental health or illness in various ways and formulate treatments based on their unique conceptualizations of both causes and cures (Heelas and Lock 1981; Jorm et al. 1997; Sue and Sue 1999) and attitudes toward psychological disorders and services among various ethnic groups can play a key role in determining utilization rates (Chiu 2004; Flum 1998; Uomoto and Gorsuch 1984). In the same way attitudes among religious groups toward psychological disorders also impact admission of problems, help-seeking behaviors, beliefs concerning aetiology and mental health utilization rates (Lafuze, Perkins and Avirappattu 2002; McClure 1987; McKindley-Alverez 2003; Roberts 1984; Taetzsch 1986). Trice and Bjorck (2006) in their study of Pentecostal perspectives on depression note that belief in divine healing (supernatural intervention by God to heal people from disease) has been a central tenet of faith and praxis (Chappel 1988).

Because primary dependence on God is emphasized during times of sickness (Murray 1982), attitudes toward doctors and medications are mixed at best (Griffith 1998; MacNutt 1988). Grant Wacker (2001) in *Heaven Below* notes how Pentecostals have always negotiated the tension between a robust belief in faith healing, which repudiated medical technology entirely, and the belief that faith healing and the use of medicine were indeed compatible. He points out that physicians were found attending early Pentecostal revival services and even participating as members in Pentecostal communities of faith. Over the generations, both the upward social mobility of many Pentecostals and their medical missionary emphases led to an increasing acceptance of the use of medicine.

Trice and Bjorck remark that Pentecostalism has historically embraced antipathy between religion and psychology (Bobgan and Bobgan 1979). Some Pentecostals may be wary of psychological treatments; some clergy believe that if psychological interventions compete with spiritual interventions, they may discourage their parishioners from seeking help from secular sources (Edwards et al. 1999).

## Pentecostalism as a Healing Movement

Healing is one of the most constant activities in the history of Christianity. As historian Amanda Porterfield (2005) explains, Jesus himself performed many miracles of healing; these acts of healing were often accompanied by forgiveness of sins (Acts 3:16). The healing in the gospels is a "sign" to prove Jesus' divinity and to foster belief in him as the Christ (John 6:2). Ideas about health and healing in Christianity have always reflected wider theological concerns and practices of healing are closely aligned to religious authority, church structure, ideas about sanctity, history, resurrection and the Kingdom of God. However, it is important to note that there are significant differences in belief about miraculous healing even among people within the same denomination in the Anglican tradition; positive belief in faith healing—healing through spiritual means—is mainly a characteristic of conservative Christians, most especially those with Charismatic experience (Village 2005).

Csordas (1988) notes that the curious blend of premodern, modern and postmodern elements in the spirit-filled worldview led to a holistic perspective on healing. Healing involves a deepening of one's relationship with God, out of which flows the secondary benefits of improved physical and emotional health. From its inception Pentecostalism has emphasized the power of the Holy Spirit to heal both physically and psychologically. Dayton (1996) emphasizes that "divine healing" was important to the development of "classical Pentecostalism" because it evidenced the "supernatural gifts of the Spirit." Griffith (1998) notes that in American Pentecostalism during the late 19th century, this promise of happiness and lack of suffering took on the added dimension of an expectation of freedom from disease and a life of vigorous health.

As Cox (2011) remarks, Pentecostals maintain that God is just as interested in our bodies on this earth, in their health and well-being, as he is in salvation for the next life. In her overview of *Global Pentecostal and Charismatic Healing*, Candy Gunther Brown (2011) asserts that Pentecostalism is more than a religious movement that emphasizes healing, but healing is central to the movement. Divine healing is the essential marker of the global phenomenon of Pentecostal and charismatic Christianity. For her, divine healing and not speaking in tongues is the single most characteristic feature of global Pentecostal and Charismatic Christianity.

The Pew Survey *Spirit and Power: A 10-Country Survey of Pentecostals* (Pew Forum on Religion & Public Life 2006) singles out healing as distinguishing Pentecostals and Charismatics from other Christians. In the US, 62 percent of Pentecostals claimed experience of healing and in one survey, 80 percent of Americans believe in the possibility of divine healing. In every country surveyed, seven out of ten had witnessed healing of illness or injury. In Asia, Africa and South America, 80 to 90 percent of first-generation Christians attribute their conversions to healing. As Belcher and Hall (2001) note, here are no creeds or formal rules within the Pentecostal movement about the practice of healing. Lack of clearly defined creeds, rules and guidelines for practice is "normative" for the movement and healing practices vary between churches. Despite these findings, there has been little attention given to these healings in different cultural contexts.

Illness is often understood by Pentecostals to be the result of demonic activity and therefore exorcism, deliverance (freeing from oppression rather than focusing on demons themselves) and healing go closely hand in hand. For practitioners of divine healing, the amelioration of physical and psychological distress is not perceived in isolation but holistically as one of the diving gifts included in "full salvation" alongside forgiveness from sin, deliverance from demonic oppression and baptism with the Holy Spirit. Healing is an important factor, as Cox (2011) rightly asserts, in drawing people to the movement and also for its widespread appeal and spread.

**Healing, Narrative and Experience**

Gunther Brown (2011) remarks that Pentecostal healing relates to an entire range of diseases: physical, mental and social. While claims are made that persons and communities experience healing from physical diseases like cancer, they also allegedly experience deliverance and healing from the diseases of poverty, joblessness and racism. Divine healing—according to Pentecostals—can heal any illness whatsoever, be it a small ailment (e.g., a headache), a mental problem (such as depression) or very serious physical maladies (e.g., cancer, AIDS, dementia). It is held to be more powerful than biomedical healing: "If you have cancer of the stomach, the doctor can remove half your insides, which may get rid of the problem, but it's not wholeness. If you go to Jesus and He heals you, you still have your stomach and you are completely restored too" (Andrews 2003). Pentecostal healing is always the work of God and the Holy Spirit, never of the person praying for healing and can be divided up into a number of components (Warrington 2006). First and foremost is "spiritual healing." In the Pentecostal movement, healing "works" first and foremost as a spiritual experience, physical and social-emotional healing are hoped for but are secondary aspects. The key element is becoming closer to God. It is the removal of perceived barriers to divine intimacy including personal sin and demonic influence, as Poloma (1998) notes, that constitutes "spiritual healing." John Wimber, a Charismatic pastor and one of the founders of the Vineyard movement, states:

The healing of our spirit, in which our relationship with God is renewed and restored, is the most fundamental area of healing. Without doubt the healing of our spirit is the lynchpin around which all other areas of healing revolve. [Wimber and Springer 1987:66]

In a second form of healing—inner healing—there is self-acceptance, healing of emotions and healing of relationships with others. Also referred to as the healing of memories or emotional healing, it is the process by which the Holy Spirit restores health to the deepest areas of an individual's life dealing with the root cause of emotional distress and pain. Williams (2013) traces Pentecostals' and Charismatics' increasing acceptance of mental forms of healing associated with psychology and the New Thought tradition. Among Charismatics, Agnes Sanford, one of the principal founders of the inner healing movement and author of *The Inner Light*, was especially influential in the formation of ministries of inner healing. Through her and her successors, for example Ruth Carter Stapleton and Francis MacNutt, many adherents in the Pentecostal–Charismatic movement were taught basic psychological principles and teachings regarding the power of visualization. While individuals who closely identified with traditional Pentecostalism often resisted inner healing practitioners' efforts to combine divine healing with psychology, even proponents of Word of Faith emphases who stressed the power of positive confession similarly cited the mind as central to the healing process. He remarks that some of the most successful Christian ministries at the turn of the 21st century have successfully combined Word of Faith themes with the spiritualized forms of popular psychology associated with US therapeutic culture.

Discernment—the ability to discern the presence of evil spirits or other causes of illness—is important for Pentecostal healing. As Thomas (1998) observes of Jesus, "He is not only able to detect when the presence of individual sin is behind an infirmity (John 5:14) but is also able to discern when this is not the case (John 9:3, Luke 13:1–5)." The ability to discern is linked by Pentecostals to the gift of prophecy; it is a gift and is not something in which one receives training. The gift of discerning of spirits is held to operate not in the human mind, but on the level of spiritual intuition. On occasion the person ministering will become suddenly aware of the name, number or nature of the evil spirits that are controlling or troubling the oppressed person and be empowered with authority to command that the sufferer be released. It is a direct revelation; as with "words" of wisdom and knowledge, it is a partial sharing of God's omniscience. It is normal practice in Pentecostal circles for the discerning of a spirit to lead to exorcising it.

Another emotional healing strategy which is found in Pentecostalism is the expression of an individual's testimony—the description of their life before salvation. These testimonies often contain elements of emotional and social struggle. The salvation experience can free them from their past life—leaving behind their old self and becoming a new person in Christ. There may however be backsliding—a tendency to revert to previous behaviors. Belcher and Hall (2001) note how the "healing" that many Pentecostals experience is often marked by periods of stability, with some periodic decompensation. But for many Pentecostals the process of "healing" may result in psychological growth.

How do Pentecostals themselves assess the authenticity of healing? Throughout its history there has been ambivalence expressed towards the use of medical documentation and its focus on objectivity to establish the authenticity of healing. In some cases, medical proof, i.e., confirmation by doctors, has been deployed as an apologetic strategy using power of biomedicine to demonstrate that healing has in fact occurred. While notable Charismatic leaders such as Kathryn Kuhlman and Oral Roberts recruited medical allies in an attempt to authenticate their healings, those skeptics outside the movement similarly used medical evidence (or its lack) to disprove their truth claims.

In other instances Pentecostals have been wary of deploying this strategy of medical documentation arguing that it indicates lack of faith. Since the 1990s Pentecostals have largely backed away from an earlier interest in medical documentation. Instead, adopting a postmodern identity that esteems both science and spiritual experience, they appeal to narrative and to sensory experience such as feelings of heat, sensations akin to electricity, diminished pain and visionary experiences as "proof" of healing.

As Enlightenment thinkers, notably John Locke, esteemed sensory experience as the path through which correct ideas enter the mind, the sense of sight gained preeminence (Schmidt 2000). In contrast Pentecostal epistemology assumes a particular hierarchy of the senses in which feeling sensory input, rather than seeing, is believing (Gunther Brown 2009). Sensory experience indicates the power, presence and concern of God. Furthermore, evangelists encourage those receiving prayer to confirm their healings by trying to do something they could not do before while feeling whether it causes pain. According to John Wimber, Christians can get a word of knowledge in any one of five ways: one can feel it, know it, read it, see it or say it. However the vast majority of times that Charismatics claim to have a word of knowledge, they feel it as a sympathetic pain in their own bodies. While they may embrace medical treatment they eschew medical documentation of religious healing as superfluous and possibly dangerous to faith (Wacker 2001). In contrast, evangelical critics of Pentecostalism consider sensory experience an untrustworthy guide to truth and focus instead on biblical teachings for this purpose (Hunt, Hamilton and Walter 1997).

Another authentication strategy has been to deploy personal testimony and use the tools of social science to investigate and authenticate claims of healing and publish these studies lending further credence to healing claims. As an example, the Vineyard movement recruited social anthropologist David Lewis to conduct a large-scale study of 2,470 registrants at a conference in Harrogate, UK. The qualitative and quantitative data were subsequently published in a book *Healing Fiction, Fantasy or Fact* (Lewis 1989). In a similar way the Toronto movement (known for the Toronto Blessing) became more interested in social scientific than in medical investigations of healing claims.

Few studies have been conducted on the expectations of Pentecostal healing. Generally Pentecostals are encouraged to pray for both physical healing and spiritual healing at the same time. In his work on Catholic Pentecostal healing, Csordas proposes that spiritual healing is a kind of consolation prize for those who receive no other form of healing—a hedge against the failure of healing prayer (1983:337). Gunther Brown (2011) in her study of Pentecostal offshoots of the Toronto Blessing in the US, Canada and Brazil found the reverse—those who requested healing of a physical problem did not generally experience healing of a mental, emotional or spiritual problem instead.

## Anthropological Insights on Pentecostal Healing: Embodied Experience

Recent work in anthropology of the senses suggests that sensory experience is vital in bridging the worlds of the material, social and spiritual (Porcello et al. 2010). This emerging field provides a critique to the Western rigid and word-based ocular-centric approach where sight is privileged above the other senses. While participant observation traditionally focuses upon what can be seen, proponents of this approach (e.g., Stoller 1989; Pinard 1991; Seremetakis 1994) argue that engaging other senses such as touch, smell, taste and hearing can provide new perspectives.

Up until now scholars of religion have paid relatively little attention to the body and its senses in relation to religious knowledge and experience. It is only recently that they have turned their attention to embodied religious practices (see for instance Luhrmann 2012). In a similar vein Gunther Brown (2012) asserts that scholars need to pay more attention not only to what religious practitioners do with their bodies but also to how the body feels and what tactile sensations communicate about people's environments and identities. Csordas (1992; 1997) in his work on Christian Catholic Charismatics proposes a theory of religious healing based upon bodily experience. Bodily rituals provide metaphors for desired mental and spiritual states thereby helping to produce them (Csordas 2002). Below I examine Pentecostal religious experience deploying work on ritual, embodiment and border transgression.

Anthropologists have asked: what are the characteristic features of this charisma of healing and prophesying? Lindhardt (2011) asserts that the distinguishing features of this variant of Christianity include formal ritual activities as well as informal, experiential and ecstatic forms of worship. God is seen as a "living fact" rather than as an object of belief. He examines Pentecostal–Charismatic ritual practice in different parts of the world, highlighting, among other things, the crucial role of ritual in creating religious communities and identities. He suggests that Pentecostals themselves may be reluctant to deploy the term ritual in a movement which emphasizes informality and spontaneity. The latter is itself closely tied to authenticity and is seen as "true" communication with God. Spontaneity is a fundamental criterion, as Csordas (1997) notes, for manifestations and experiences of the sacred. The term ritual for many Pentecostals connotes formalism and invariance and is associated with formal, prescribed and empty liturgy; they maintain that too much doctrine impedes God's interventions and movements. For the same reasons anthropologists may have eschewed ritual theory with its similar emphasis on formalism (e.g., Bloch 1974). Scholars such as Robbins (2001) however argue that we should not be informed by these emic uses of the term ritual and that it does indeed make sense to see many Pentecostal–Charismatic cooperative and spiritually oriented activities as rituals.

Lindhardt (2011) moves away from the traditional anthropological preoccupation with ritual as symbolic enactment and discusses how rituals create new embodied orientations towards the world among practitioners, i.e., how rituals do what they do, rather than focus on just what they do. This occurs through music, song, prayer, swaying and other kinesthetic and rhythmic movements of the body. Music embraces worshipers, ushering them into God's presence. Sitting, according to him, facilitates appropriation of intellectual truths while standing and oscillatory movements facilitate engagement with experiential truths. Through a process of absorption distinctions between the self and outside environment, stimulus and response become blurred and the sense of individual self vanishes.

Moving on to boundaries, as Luedke and West (2006) note, transgression of borders is vital for religious healing generally, both in a literal sense (in terms of healers crossing the nation-state borders, borders between the local and the urban, the national and the global, etc.) but also in a more symbolic sense of crossing borders between the material and the invisible supernatural world. The extant literature from Africa on Pentecostalism points to the importance of this latter border, of the openness of Pentecostalism not only to the spiritual but also to the occult. Meyer (1999) observed in her analyses of Ewe Christians in Ghana that early missionaries appealed to the devil in order to make a boundary between what was Christian and what was "heathen." The devil, denoting the ancestral spirits and gods, was not seen by the missionaries as a real power in the world, thus creating an absolute border. The Pentecostal churches that gained popularity in the 1980s in Ghana challenged this border and began again to take the devil seriously. The Charismatic space in these Pentecostal churches thus challenged these absolute borders between the material and the invisible forces, between the good and the bad, between the old spirits and the new spirits. This porousness of the border between the occult and Christianity has been called "ontological ambivalence" (Smith 2001). While on the one hand, there is an outspoken battle against the occult forces in the Pentecostal churches, on the other hand, these forces are thereby becoming more emphasized and more powerfully present (Eriksen 2014). As Engelke (2010) notes regarding the African context, this break with the past is often ambivalent; the break is always also realignment with the past. Furthermore the break effectively makes the past more visible; the ancestral spirits increase their presence in the very effort to break with them. The Charismatic space described in the Pentecostalism literature thus appears to be characterized by a fundamental attempt to challenge borders.

While the literature on Pentecostalism has paid attention to the local and the global, little attention has been devoted to the spatial aspects of healing. Krause (2014:43) asserts that "space is about the simultaneous incorporation into a globe spanning Christian movement and the personal intimate encounter with God." The person looking for healing has to get rid of evil spirits, themselves perceived to be local and specific, and instead to become filled with the Holy Spirit whose geographical location is delocalized and unmarked in contrast to these evil spirits. There is a tension between marked and unmarked spatiality. For her the global and local, rather than being "out there," are actively produced in Pentecostal practice and teaching. Being "born again" can be seen as conversion to the global, thus leaving behind the sinful local tradition.

In relation to space, she analyzed different spatial practices related to Pentecostal healing among Pentecostal believers who migrated from Ghana to London, UK. She specifically explored the relationship between space and the manifestation of the Holy Spirit by looking at how points of contact with the divine are created in the personal life of people and at the sites where the casting out of demons takes place. Unlike in other spirit-centered healing traditions, the Christian Holy Spirit was not conceived of as embodied in specific places, but rather is spatially unbound.

## Conclusion

This chapter has examined the role of healing in the Pentecostal movement. It has argued that the provision of healing has played a significant part in its growth and worldwide popularity. There has been a move among some Pentecostal groups to abandon medical documentation and deploy bodily experiences to validate healing. This move towards phenomenological experience has significant implications for future research in this area. There is a need for detailed phenomenological accounts of healing experiences particularly the description of bodily sensations, moods, visions, voices and the ways they are interpreted and contested both by the individuals experiencing them and by the wider Pentecostal community and how they are attributed to the Holy Spirit. These aims require in-depth ethnographic interviews alongside focused participant observation. Recent phenomenological work in anthropology of religion on hearing God's voice (Luhrmann 2012) provides an excellent example of how this can be done. Although not specifically dealing with healing, Luhrmann examines how evangelical Christians in the US learn to concentrate upon their inner experiences to hear God and make the Holy Spirit "really real." Her text illustrates the emerging trend in anthropology of religion towards phenomenological approaches and a similar methodology can be deployed to examine Pentecostal healing.

## Notes

Empirical research on Pentecostalism and health has focused on two areas: the prevalence of psychiatric disorders among Pentecostals (Belcher and Hall 2001; Castelein 1984; Gritzmacher, Bolton and Dana 1998; Koenig et al. 1994; Meador et al. 1992; Poloma 1989; Pattison and Casey 1969), and the efficacy of religious healing in relation to one specific Pentecostal experience—the Toronto Blessing (Poloma 2003). I shall not develop these themes here.

## References

Andrews, I. 2003 Equipped to Heal. Columbus, GA: TEC Publications.

Barker, I. V. 2005 Engendering Charismatic Economies: Pentecostalism, Global Political Economy, and the Crisis of Social Reproduction. Paper presented at the annual meeting of the American Political Science Association, Washington, DC, September 1.

Barrett, D., and T. Johnson 2004 Annual Statistical Table on Global Mission. International Bulletin of Missionary Research 28:24–25.

Belcher, J. R., and S. M. Hall 2001 Healing and Psychotherapy. Pastoral Psychology 50:65–75.

Bloch, M. 1974 Symbols, Song, Dance and Features of Articulation: Is Religion an Extreme Form of Authority? Archives Européenes de Sociologie 15:55–81.

Bobgan, D., and M. Bobgan 1979 The Psychological Way/the Spiritual Way. Minneapolis: Bethany Fellowship.

Castelein, J. D. 1984 Glossolalia and the Psychology of the Self and Narcissism. Journal of Religion and Health 23:47–62.

Chappel, P. 1988 Healing Movements. *In* Dictionary of Pentecostal and Charismatic Movements. S. Burgess and G. McGee, eds. Pp. 363–374. Grand Rapids, MI: Zondervan.

Chiu, M. 2004 Why Chinese Women Do Not Seek Help: A Cultural Perspective on the Psychology of Women. Counseling Psychology Quarterly 17:155–166.

Cox, H. 2011 Foreword. *In* Global Pentecostal and Charismatic Healing. C. Gunther Brown, ed. Pp. xvii–xxi. New York: Oxford University Press.

Csordas, T. J. 1983 The Rhetoric of Transformation in Ritual Healing. Culture, Medicine and Psychiatry 7(4):333–375.

———. 1988 Elements of Charismatic Persuasion and Healing. Medical Anthropology Quarterly 2:121–142.

———. 1992 The Affliction of Martin: Religious, Clinical and Phenomenological Meaning in a Case of Demonic Oppression. *In* Ethnopsychiatry: The Cultural Construction of Professional and Folk Psychiatry. A. D. Gaines, ed. Pp. 125–170. Albany: State University of New York Press.

———. 1997 Language, Charisma and Creativity: The Ritual Life of a Religious Movement. Berkeley: University of California Press.

———. 2002 Body/Meaning/Healing. New York: Palgrave Macmillan.

Dayton, D. W. 1996 Theological Roots of Pentecostalism. Peabody, MA: Hendrickson Publishers.

Dobbins, R. 2000 Psychotherapy with Pentecostal Protestants. *In* Handbook of Psychotherapy and Religious Diversity. P. Richards and A. Bergin, eds. Pp. 155–184. Washington, DC: American Psychological Association.

Edwards, L., B. Lim, M. McMinn, and A. Dominguez 1999 Examples of Collaboration between Psychologists and Clergy. Professional Psychology: Research and Practice 30:547–551.

Engelke, M. 2010 Past Pentecostalism: Notes on Rupture, Realignment, and Everyday Life in Pentecostal and African Independent Churches. Africa 80(2):177–199.

Eriksen, A. 2014 Sarah's Sinfulness: Egalitarianism, Denied Difference, and Gender in Pentecostal Christianity. Current Anthropology 55(S10):S262–S270.

Flum, M. E. 1998 Attitudes toward Mental Health and Help-Seeking Preferences of Chinese, Japanese and Korean International College Students. Dissertation Abstracts International 59 (1470).

Griffith, R. 1998 "Joy Unspeakable and Full of Glory": The Vocabulary of Pious Emotion in the Narratives of American Pentecostal Women,

1910–1940. *In* An Emotional History of the United States. P. Stearns and J. Lewis, eds. Pp. 218–240. New York: New York University Press.

Gritzmacher, S. A., B. Bolton, and R. H. Dana 1998 Psychological Characteristics of Pentecostals: A Literature Review and Psycho-Dynamic Synthesis. Journal of Psychology and Theology 16:233–245.

Gunther Brown, C. 2009 Touch and American Religions. Religion Compass 3(4):770–783.

———. 2011 Global Pentecostal and Charismatic Healing. Oxford: Oxford University Press.

Hammond, F., and I. M. Hammond 2010 [1973] Pigs in the Parlor: The Practical Guide to Deliverance. Kirkwood, MO: Impact Christian Books.

Heelas, P., and A. Lock, eds. 1981 Indigenous Psychologies: The Anthropology of the Self. London: Academic Press.

Hunt, S., M. Hamilton, and T. Walter, eds. 1997 Charismatic Christianity: Sociological Perspectives. New York: St. Martin's Press.

Jorm, A., A. Korten, P. Jacomb, H. Christensen, B. Rodgers, and P. Pollitt 1997 Public Beliefs about Causes and Risk Factors for Depression and Schizophrenia. Social Psychiatry and Psychiatric Epidemiology 32:143–148.

Koenig, H. G., L. K. George, K. G. Meador, D. G. Blazer, and P. B. Dyck 1994 Religious Affiliation and Psychiatric Disorder among Protestant Baby Boomers. Hospital and Community Psychiatry 45:586–596.

Krause, K. 2014 Space in Pentecostal Healing Practices among Ghanaian Migrants in London. Medical Anthropology 33(1):37–51.

Lafuze, J., D. Perkins, and G. Avirappattu 2002 Pastors' Perceptions of Mental Disorders. Psychiatric Services 53:900–901.

Lewis, D. 1989 Healing: Fiction, Fantasy, or Fact? London: Hodder & Stoughton Religious.

Lindhardt, M., ed. 2011 Practicing the Faith: The Ritual Life of Pentecostal–Charismatic Christians. New York: Berghahn.

Luedke, T. J., and H. G. West 2006 Introduction—Healing Divides: Therapeutic Border Work in Southeast Africa. *In* Borders and Healers: Brokering Therapeutic Resources in Southeast Africa. T. J. Luedke and H. G. West, eds. Pp. 1–20. Bloomington, IN: Indiana University Press.

Luhrmann, T. 2012 When God Talks Back: Understanding the American Evangelical Relationship with Prayer. New York: Knopf.

MacNutt, F. 1988 Healing. Alamonte Springs, FL: Creation House.

McClure, R. 1987 Religion, Admission of Emotional Problems, and Seeking Therapeutic Help. Psychology: A Journal of Human Behavior 24:33–36.

McKindley-Alverez, C. 2003 African American Baptists' Attitudes toward Psychotherapy. Dissertation Abstracts International 64 (1500B).

Meador, K., H. Koenig, D. Hughes, D. Blazer, J. Turnbull, and L. George 1992 Religious Affiliation and Major Depression. Hospital and Community Psychology 43:1204–1208.

Meyer, B. 1999 Translating the Devil: Religion and Modernity and the Ewe in Ghana. Edinburgh: Edinburgh University Press.

Murray, A. 1982 Divine Healing. Springdale, PA: Whitaker House.

Pattison, E. M., and R. L. Casey 1969 Glossolalia: A Contemporary Mystical Experience. Clinical Psychiatry and Religion 5:133–148.

Pew Forum on Religion & Public Life 2006 Spirit and Power: A 10-Country Survey of Pentecostals. www.pewforum.org/files/2006/10/pentecostals-08.pdf, accessed April 1, 2016.

Pinard, S. 1991 A Taste of India: On the Role of Gustation in the Hindu Sensorium. In Varieties of Sensory Experience: A Sourcebook in the Anthropology of the Senses. D. Howes, ed. Pp. 221–230. Toronto: University of Toronto Press.

Poloma, M. M. 1989 The Assemblies of God at the Crossroads: Charisma and Institutional Dilemmas. Knoxville: University of Tennessee Press.

———. 1998 The 'Toronto Blessing': A Holistic. Model of Healing. Journal for the Scientific Study of Religion 37:258–273.

———. 2003 Main Street Mystics: The Toronto Blessing and Reviving Pentecostalism. Walnut Creek, CA: AltaMira.

Porcello, T., L. Meintjes, A. M. Ochoa, and D. Samuels 2010 The Reorganization of the Sensory World. Annual Review of Anthropology 39:51–56.

Porterfield, A. 2005 Healing in the History of Christianity. Oxford: Oxford University Press.

Robbins, J. 2001 Introduction: Global Religions, Pacific Island Transformations. Journal of Ritual Studies 15(2):7–12.

Roberts, C. 1984 Current Conservative Religious Attitudes towards Seeking Professional Counselling. Dissertation Abstracts International 55 (09A).

Ruthven, J. 1997 On the Cessation of the Charismata: The Protestant Polemic on Post-Biblical Miracles. Sheffield: Sheffield Academic Press.

Schmidt, L. E. 2000 Hearing Things: Religion, Illusion, and the American Enlightenment. Cambridge: Harvard University Press.

Seremetakis, C. N. 1994 The Memory of the Senses, Part I: Marks of the Transitory. *In* The Senses Still: Memory and Perception as Material Culture in Modernity. C. N. Seremetakis, ed. Pp. 1–18. Boulder: Westview Press.

Smith, D. J. 2001 "The Arrow of God": Pentecostalism, Inequality, and the Supernatural in South-Eastern Nigeria. Africa 71(4):587–613.

Stoller, P. 1989 The Taste of Ethnographic Things: The Senses in Anthropology. Philadelphia: University of Pennsylvania Press.

Sue, D. W., and D. Sue 1999 Counseling the Culturally Different: Theory and Practice. New York: Wiley.

Taetzsch, W. J. 1986 The Orientation of Evangelical Christians toward Seeking Psychotherapy. Dissertation Abstracts International 47 (6B).

Thiessen, H. 1979 Lectures in Systematic Theology. Grand Rapids: Eerdmans.

Thomas, J. C. 1998 The Devil, Disease and Deliverance: Origins of Illness in New Testament Thought. Sheffield: Sheffield Academic Press.

Trice, P. D., and J. P. Bjorck 2006 Pentecostal Perspectives on Causes and Cures of Depression. Professional Psychology: Research and Practice 37(3):283–294.

Uomoto, J., and R. Gorsuch 1984 Japanese American Response to Psychological Disorder: Referral Patterns, Attitudes, and Subjective Norms. American Journal of Community Psychology 12:537–550.

Village, A. 2005 Dimensions of Belief about Miraculous Healing. Mental Health, Religion & Culture 8(2):97–107.

Wacker, G. 2001 Heaven Below: Early Pentecostals and American Culture. Cambridge: Harvard University Press.

Warrington, K. 2006 Healing Matters: Jesus' Powerful Pointers. Direction 54:30–31.

Williams, J. 2013 Minding the Spirit in Spirit Cure: A History of Pentecostal Healing. Oxford: Oxford University Press.

Wimber, J., and K. Springer 1987 Power Healing. San Francisco: Harper & Row.

# Chapter 11

## Tradition, Emotion, Healing and the Sacred: Revivalist Lamenting in Finland in Relation to Three Authenticities

*James M. Wilce*

### Introduction and Background

The tripartite theme of religion, healing and psychiatry is one of great interest, and this volume has the potential to contribute to each of the themes, and to the theoretical agendas of fields like anthropology more generally. This chapter addresses lament, and more specifically Karelian (and "neo-Karelian") lament across a transformative century. People at both ends of this time period have regarded lament as *pyhä* or "sacred," while conceiving of its sacredness in radically different ways. The sacredness of lament in 19$^{th}$ century Karelia and contemporary Finland has everything to do with healing and even psychiatry (or more properly, the psy-disciplines [Rose 1996], which include psychology and various forms of counseling/therapy as well as psychiatry).[1] By this I mean that lament (for instance, funeral lament), which was once practiced as a means of helping the dead soul in its journey to the other world, has become something very different in its new incarnation in the so-called lament revival in Finland. Lamenting has become a self-healing practice—one among many other such practices in postmodern Finland.

In this essay I concentrate on the lament "revival," the organization *Äänellä Itkijät* (Those Who Cry With Voice/Words), hereafter referred to as ÄI-Lamenters, and their "Healing Lament" courses. Finland has witnessed an explosion of spiritual healing modalities designatable as "New Age" (though not without profound controversy) or as "post-secular" (Utriainen, Broo and Hovi 2012). Picking and choosing elements from disparate traditions is a feature of post-secular spiritualities, and contemporary Finnish lamenting exemplifies that tendency. Finnish courses in

---

[1] Nikolas Rose (1996:2) uses "psy-" as shorthand for "the psychosciences and disciplines—psychology, psychiatry, and their cognates."

lament (wept song, tuneful weeping with words) combine lessons from the tradition of sacred lament in Karelia (a region some Finns regard as their cultural heartland) with healing conceived along psychotherapeutic lines (i.e., reflecting the influence of the "psy-disciplines" psychiatry, psychology, social work, etc., [Rose 1996]).

Of all the places in the world where lament has thrived, then disappeared, it is remarkable that the Finnish region would be the one to host a revival. The irony lies in the stereotype—spread by Finns themselves, inter alia— that Finnish people, especially men, are unable to share their feelings. The stereotype is important in the ongoing work of the ÄI-Lamenters, for whom teaching more Finns to lament is motivated by the conviction that they desperately need such skills, that lament can be their salvation. Thus, what may seem to be an odd and marginal example of post-Christian proselytizing is to revivalists the most important thing they can do. Still, their outreach (especially to Finnish men) is an uphill battle.

Beyond describing lament and its function in the Finnish region, this essay theorizes "healing lament" vis-à-vis notions of authenticity, and particularly three concepts of "authenticity" emerging in lament courses. The first, which I call "cultural-replicative authenticity," entails a claim that one lament replicates enough of the exact words and actions of previous laments to be considered a shoot from the same cultural branch. "Previous" and "current" laments could mean either a pair of "traditional" laments or a traditional performance compared with a lament that is modern yet contains enough traditional features to be judged an authentic replication.

It is the second form of authenticity—the personal-expressive—that Trilling treats in his groundbreaking work (1972). Trilling says authenticity is not "sincerity," the latter being exemplified by Polonius' statement in Hamlet that "if one is true to oneself, one can be false to no other" (as cited by Trilling 1972:9). Both sincerity and personal authenticity involve being honest or providing an accurate reflection of one's inner being. But our contemporaries in the "Age of Authenticity" ask, "If one is true to one's own self for the purpose of avoiding falsehood to others, is one being true to one's own self?" (Trilling 1972:9). Unlike sincerity, personal-expressive authenticity is an obligation to oneself, for the sake of oneself. We see the quest to be true to oneself for its own sake in cultural practices and understandings. Today, "we want to discover and express our essential selves in rapturous church services, in charged therapy sessions, in risky sports, in intense personal relationships" (Lindholm 2008:65). Modern laments seek to channel "personal-expressive" authenticity, although "cultural authenticity" also exerts a pull on neo-lamenting.

I refer to the third form of authenticity as "spirit-relational"—rather than "ritually efficacious," for example—because (1) efficacy is at stake in all three forms of authenticity, and (2) the efficacy of this third form is culturally understood as a reflection of a lamenter's relationship with (i.e., to speak to) spirits. Finally, (3) labeling this third form "spirit-relational" engages Lau's important work on authenticities. It is an adaptation of Lau's "relationship authenticity." Whereas for Lau this form of authenticity entails honest sharing in interpersonal relationships (2010), I use "spirit-relational" to denote authentication of a performance based on complex signs adding up to "efficacy," which in turn reflects a relationship with the more-than-human. Traditional Karelian laments were largely judged according to such spiritual-relational criteria as their aftereffects—i.e., their magical power.

To explicate these models of authenticity and their relationship to the therapeutic-*cum*-sacred quality of modern Finnish lament courses I draw on semiotics and particularly theories of metasemiotic representation. It is important to note at this point, however, that it may well be more accurate to speak of three distinct authenticities, or even three distinct frames, each of which invokes a unique metadiscourse that legitimates or otherwise empowers some object, object–sign or set of relations that becomes the object of reflection.

This chapter explores the emergence of multiple authenticities at semiotic crossroads where ideological formulations of relationships between *itkuvirsi* and the semiotic objects that anchor lament's authenticity meet distinctions between performance and performativity. In various ways, social actors draw on and combine these rich semiotic resources either to stake their claims to authenticity or to challenge those made by others.

We start by suggesting the inherently relational nature of authenticity such that, to consider something as authentic involves framing it as related in a particular way (a Peircean "ground") to something else (a Peircean "object") (Hanks 1996). The sign-object may be an objectifiable entity (a thing or practice) external to that something (an authentic example of

*Wilce*

x, or even an authentic replica of x, as in Bruner [1994]), or a quality of either the experience of that something (Wang 1999), or the context of its emergence (Bruner 1994). "Authenticity" is a metasemiotic term that comments on the sorts of relationships described in the foregoing paragraph.

**Authentic With Regard To What? Authenticity and Its Externalities**

In its earliest recorded uses in English—as with its forerunners in French, Latin and Greek—the label "authentic" (*authentik*) presupposed, but also performatively created, links between features of a particular text and conventionally agreed-upon features of an *Ur*-text. To call something authentic was thus to guarantee its authority vis-à-vis externalities.[2] Therefore, the authentic bore a certain relationship to something, and granting something authenticity involved an external process of legitimation. In that vein, exemplified by Asplund's rejection of Martta Kuikka's lament, the authenticity of neolament performance may be made to depend on its replication of a particular traditional lament by a "master."[3]

Yet, in our post- or late modern age such an objectivizing use is neither the only nor the central use. In many influential explorations, a personal, subjective authenticity has become so salient that it appears to be the only form worth contemplating. For example, in dubbing ours the "Age of Authenticity," Taylor (2007)—like Trilling (1972) before him—betrays no interest in authenticities other than one definable as "being true to self for self's sake." Does this mean, however, that such forms of authenticity do not rely on externalities? While the "authentic self" of subjective authenticity could be argued to have escaped the need of any external anchoring for its validation—after all, it is you and I who know whether this is our true selves shining through—the apparent escape is illusory. While the authenticity of the self may seem to be unmoored from an external object as a measure of its verisimilitude, it still answers to external crite-

---

[2] Authenticity's etymological tendency toward an external orientation is indicated in the phrase "of established credit" in the *Oxford English Dictionary* definition.

[3] For the use of "master" (Karelian *moast'eri*) in metasemiotic commentary about the very best lamenters, perhaps seen as a model or teacher, see Konkka (1985:107).

ria. In fact, it provides its own metasemiotic tools through which a listener (e.g., a psychotherapist) can discern the "real" from the "unreal" experience of the authentic (Smith in press). When authenticity is not anchored in a tangible, external object it is still assessed against a conceptual externality on which the Peircean "interpretant" (Harks 1996:42) can seize to pronounce x (in)authentic in relation to y at any level of semiosis. Thus, even though Wang (1999) in his discussion of existential authenticity identifies it as an activity-related, non-objectified state of being, such authenticity—while it may not rely on the authenticity of tangible objects—still hinges on an externality of sorts. It relies on understandings of what makes the experience authentic, and how we can make such determinations. If, as Deleuze notes, a Platonic "well-founded" copy (authentic in Bruner's sense of verisimilitude) "proceeds less from one thing to another than from a thing to an Idea" (1983:48), its authenticity still depends on an externality of essence or form. The authenticity of a neolament performance evaluated through its concordance with the old genre (as a faithful token of a type), rather than by its repetition or replication of a particular old lament (relating as copy-to-original), exemplifies such an anchorage in a multiplex object that may not be a tangible one but certainly is an object in the semiotic sense.

## Lament as Sacred Tradition, "Healing Lament" as Psy-Sacred Hybrid

In keeping with the dominance of a certain kind of authenticity, especially in cultural settings most profoundly influenced by Protestant Christianity,[4] "psy- has played a key role in constituting our current regime of the self" (Rose 1996:2). For a time, a form of modernization theory asserted the one-way influence of psy- on religion, politics and culture. In Finland, for example, Kivivuori (1991) asserted that *psykokulttuuri* (psychoculture) was so influential in religious groups like the Evangelical Lutheran Church of Finland that traditional (theological) understandings of salvation were giving way to a new soteriology—a theological model explaining how people are "saved." Gone was redemption from sin. Lu-

---

[4] Note that Protestant discourse prefers "sincerity" (Keane 2007) over "authenticity," for good theological reasons (given that "authenticity" involves an exaltation of the self with which many Protestant groups are uncomfortable).

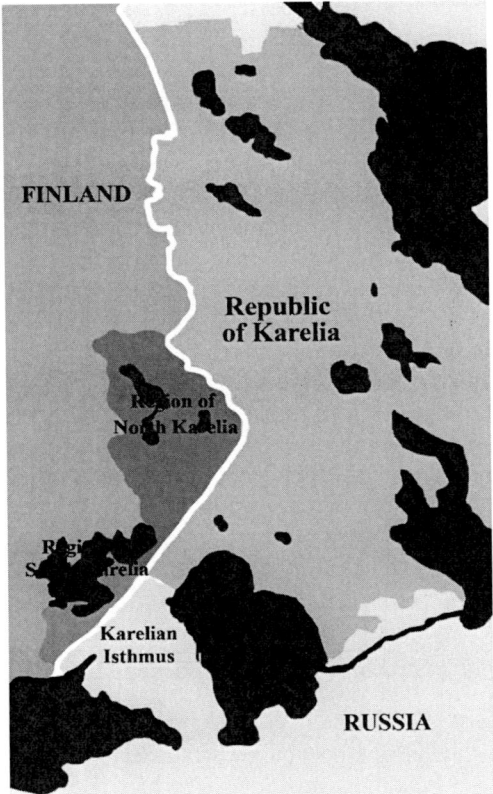

*Figure 1: Map of the Republic of Karelia.*

theranism seemed destined to become an institution devoted to personal liberation from guilt feelings. According to Utriainen (this volume; also Utriainen, Hovi and Broo 2012), the pushback by "post-secular spiritualities" in Finland is as significant as the momentum of psy-. Spiritual technologies of the self—ways of managing emotions, et cetera, by recourse to spiritual practices—are infiltrating ostensibly secular institutions.

In what follows, I introduce "traditional" Karelian lamenting and its so-called revival in contemporary lament courses. I hope to show how the two might enable us to think in new ways about religion or the sacred, healing and psychiatry, or rather the use of specifically psy-concepts in construing lament old and new.

This chapter is based on 11 months of ethnographic fieldwork in 2008 and 2009 that focused on the "lament revival" in contemporary Finland and particularly on the revivalist organization ÄI-Lamenters (introduced earlier). That fieldwork included participant observation in, and audio and video recordings of, six lament courses; interviews with 16 lament course participants (alumni) and visits to the audio archives of the Finnish Literature Society.

## Context for Contemporary Lament Courses: The History of Karelian Lament

Karelia is a stateless transnational region (Roberts 2004) straddling the border between Finland and Russia. Whereas no firm evidence indicates that western Finns have ever had their own lament tradition, smaller Finno-Ugrian groups like Karelians, Ingrians and Komis (to name but a few) had thriving lament traditions in the 19th century (Honko 1963). Lament played a vital role in rural Karelian ritual observances. There were funeral and wedding laments, as well as "recruit laments."[5] In any given village, all women knew the genre and were obliged to perform it at least at funerals if not other rituals of leave-taking.

Let us focus for a while just on funeral laments in Karelia. Upon death, improvised laments accompanied all of the steps in mortuary rituals lasting at least three days. Although all the women who gathered around the dead were obliged to lament, it was customary to invite a particularly skilled lamenter to lead the mourning. Respect for the key audiences— not only the spirit of the deceased but also ancestral spirits as key addressees of traditional lament—explains why people say that lamentation itself deserves respect. All of the many laments performed during the funeral observances not only shared but actively contributed to the sacredness of the ritual time and space (Stepanova 2011).

---

[5] Karelian village women performed "recruit laments" when a son, husband, or father was conscripted into the army. Such men were not expected to return alive.

Ritual lamentation was thus *pyhä* (sacred) and a manifestation of a power that could be both beneficent and dangerous (Koski 2008). Although the expression of grief and other emotions was very important in old Karelian laments, I find no evidence in Karelian lament scholarship (interviews, etc.) that lamenting was considered *hoitava* (healing or personally therapeutic). But "therapeutic" is exactly what ÄI-Lamenters call their practice, which is profoundly influenced by post-Freudian notions of individual emotional liberation even as it maintains its strong links to Karelian tradition.

## The Esoteric Karelian Lament Register

The obligation to lament reflected the understanding "that crying [lamenting], literally, opens the gates of Tuonela [the land of the dead in Finnic tradition]," and "that those family members who [had] died before them, upon hearing the crying, would come to greet the newly deceased" (Konkka 1985:187).[6] Although Karelian laments were improvised, they also adhered to traditional performance forms, particularly to that set of linguistic features that villagers accepted as the language (technically, the specialized linguistic register [Agha 2007]) of the deceased, the ancestors who joined the living at ritual moments and various deities. In using the *itkukieli* or "lament register," lamenters felt that they were communicatively acting with, upon and for these beings.

Compared with their neighbors, highly skilled lamenters had the strongest grasp of the lament register. Its lexical features included a list of roughly 1,400 of the sort of canonical "circumlocutions," fixed phrases that enabled lamenters to avoid direct mention of a whole range of people and common things in their environment (Stepanova 2011). A lamenter who is properly avoiding any direct mention of the deceased by kin name ("mother") might say "oh thou who carried me into the world" (Pirkko Fihlman, personal communication, April 2009). These lamenters' special grasp of the register, and their role in helping the dead find their way to the afterworld, justifies referring to them as psychopomps (Tolbert 1990), although—unlike their counterparts in Greek mythology—these women

---

[6] The quoted material comes from the Russian summary of Konkka's Finnish-language account of Karelian lament, as translated by Janina Fenigsen (2012), to whom I am most grateful.

did not accompany the *vainajat* (souls of the deceased) on their journey. Instead, their wept songs themselves somehow did the guiding.

All who gathered for traditional Karelian funerals—family, neighbors, friends and invited lamenters—were expected to demonstrate certain emotions, including grief over the *vainaja* and respect not only for the departed but other classes of spirits gathered for the ritual (ancestors and lesser deities). The enactments, around the time of death, of the aforementioned emotions, including the emotions shown by the kind of skilled lamenters invited to funerals, were culturally normative.

People often talk about norms. No doubt Karelian villagers, right up through the 20th century, openly discussed particular laments, and lamentation in general. And given what we know about "emotion regimes" (Reddy 2001; Wilce 2009) around the world and across history, it is unlikely that Karelian metasemiotic comments concerned the extent to which external expression of grief matched internal experience. Neither family members nor invited lamenters were necessarily concerned about one another's sincerity (truth for others' sake) or authenticity (personal-expressive authenticity, being true to oneself for one's own sake [Trilling 1972]). Instead, community members probably judged lamenters' performances in relationship to the first and third authenticities. They probably weighed the extent to which the lament reproduced discursive conventions. Evidence indicates that the skilled lamenter's powerful emotions were taken to be signs of a kind of trance possession in which the lamenter took on the role of a "female shaman" (Tolbert 1990), demonstrating not (or not just) "personal" but (also) "spirit-relational" authenticity.

## The Finnish "Lament Revival," the Organization Leading It, and Lament Courses

Understanding lament courses offered by ÄI-Lamenters requires some comparison with other such courses in Finland—other lament courses but also radically different "healing" courses. Other courses with which I am familiar enshrine different notions of personhood and healing; for example, some lack any emphasis on "psy-" or personal authenticity. ÄI-Lament courses stand out insofar as no other "healing" course includes (1) music, weeping, words governed by "local" cultural tradition, (2) intense

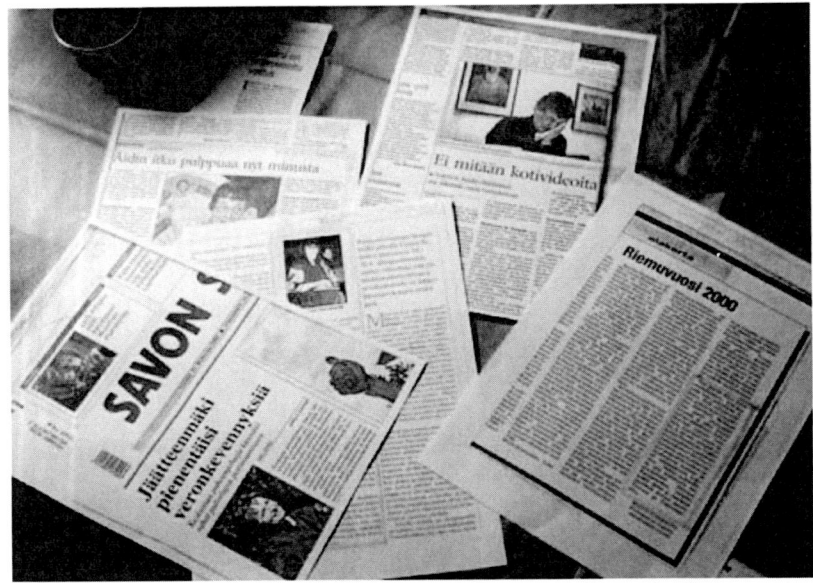

*Figure 2: Newspaper articles covering a lamenter from the Savo region, who collected them over a long period of time.*

media attention provoking fairly widespread metadiscourse, (3) appeal to a "psy-ready" constituency or (4) a sacred function.

Concepts of authenticity hold the keys to understanding precisely how religion, healing and psychiatry come together in the practice of lamenting in Karelia and Finland. And key to the understanding of authenticity is grasping the relationship between signs and metasigns, practice (e.g., lamenting) and reflection (e.g., judging a lament authentic or inauthentic vis-à-vis some model).

Various figures active in Finland's lament "revival" have disagreed over the goals and methods of lament courses. Is lamenting all about self-help, or is it a performance of a sacred cultural practice? If it is the latter, then neo-Karelian lament must faithfully reproduce the semiotic forms and functions constituting traditional lament. If lamenting is a mode of self-healing, then anything that gets in the way—including "excessive" concern for replicating old forms such as the circumlocutions—is undesirable. These differences over the proper linguistic forms to use in lamenting correlate with divergent notions of its function and sacredness.

Traditional Karelian laments were, of course, performed in the Karelian language, but neolamenters gathering in Finland for intimate lament courses (consisting of no more than ten participants) sing in Finnish. None of the leaders of various branches of the "lament revival" requires performance in the Karelian language. Still, all of them commend to their students some features of the traditional lament register. The most traditionally oriented of contemporary Finnish lamenters advocates use of alliteration and verbatim Finnish counterparts of the 1,400 Karelian-language circumlocutions. Her understanding of lament's sacredness has nothing to do with what ÄI-Lamenters emphasize (healing, authentic self-expression or the achievement of intimacy based on such "sharing"). For her as for her ancestors, the sacrality of traditional laments reflects their use in communicating with sacred entities. Since this "traditionalist" is less concerned with personal authenticity and healing through lament and has taught somewhat fewer lament courses than her counterparts in ÄI-Lamenters, I focus on ÄI.

ÄI-Lamenters have taught roughly 2,000 Finns since their founding in 2001. They encourage students to invent their own "metaphors" or "pictorial language." They advertise their courses as a way to experience *Hoitava Itku* (Healing Lament). Their teaching links the "healing power of laments" to their "personal-expressive authenticity," in a manner reminiscent of various courses in the US that teach participants how to feel and express their feelings, and even to experience group emotional encounters as sacred (Holloman 1974; Heelas 1981).

Who attends Finnish lament courses? ÄI-Lament course participants are almost all middle-class women who can afford both the time (a weekend, from Friday evening to Sunday late afternoon) and the registration fee. Despite the predominance of women, ÄI leaders profess a special concern for Finnish men, said to suffer from many problems because they "cannot" express their emotions. Courses attract women in many professions, but consistently include therapists—practitioners of art and sex therapy, psychodrama, et cetera—or those from allied professions such as psychiatric nursing. Probably some 20 percent of ÄI's trainees since 2001 have a strong Karelian background. Many have experienced either other kinds of lament classes or other New Age "healing" courses.

In the climax of my argument, later in this chapter, I provide direct evidence of what revival leaders say about lament, authenticity, healing and the sacred. First, however, I need to more thoroughly contextualize their concepts of authenticity in relation to the layers of reflection that concepts of authenticity entail.

## Authenticities

Be it in Finnish or English, we (as social actors as well as scholars) use the term "authenticity" (*aitous* in Finnish) in multiple ways. Yet "authenticity" is always a metasign, a sign that reflects on another sign. It is a word–sign that describes the relationship between some sort of second and third sign. I will concentrate on three ways in which Finns use *aitous* (authenticity)—cultural-replicative authenticity, personal-expressive authenticity and spirit-relational. To speak of something as "authentic" in the cultural sense is to invoke the connection between a contemporary performance and its predecessors. Personal authenticity involves "individuals interacting on the basis of their real selves" (Lau 2010:480), using expressive signs that perfectly reflect that emotional self which Western thought envisions as underlying the expression. Finally, "spirit-relational authenticity" requires a lamenter, for example, to produce a set of signs that indicate that she is communicating effectively with the more-than-human world, and particularly to produce an accumulation of evidence that her performance has been magically efficacious. This third authenticity was especially relevant in popular judgments of traditional lament. Although in some New Age contexts the personal-expressive authenticity competes for dominance with cultural authenticity, I see in lament courses a tense equilibrium between all three senses of authenticity.

## Metasemiotics

All societies have ways of reflecting on the signs they produce via another set of (meta)signs. Metasemiotic discourse is discourse reflecting, for instance, on all of the sign modalities that constitute a (neo)Karelian lament—the proper posture, crying-voice quality, "lyrics," et cetera. In the following section I analyze the semiotic structure involved in the three authenticities most relevant to (neo)Karelian lament.

## Three Authenticities and Their Particular Semiotic Structure

The evaluation of a set of signs as authentic in any sense is a metasemiotic activity; it involves one set of signs (discourse about authenticity) reflecting on two other sets of signs. Attempts to authenticate or de-authenticate a lament as a cultural performance and candidate for being judged culturally authentic involve

(1) some set of signs understood as a potential predecessor or model vis-à-vis another set produced later;

(2) another set whose relationship to the first set is in question and

(3) a third level of signs addressing the relationship between the first two sets of signs, the third set providing the judgment to which producers of set (2) orient their performance, judgments that construe set (2) as faithful in a fairly literal sense to sign-set (1).

The semiotic structure of the second, "personal-expressive," form of authenticity involves

(1) some set of signs understood to be interior to some social actor (e.g., emotions in and of themselves as signs—for instance, reactions to the perception of external events);

(2) another set of signs, e.g., linguistic signs, by which that social actor is understood to reveal, perform or act out the first set and

(3) a judgment by other actors that construes the relationship between (2) and (1) as transparent or opaque, true or false, authentic or inauthentic—or that intervenes in that relationship. An example of such interventions is Rogerian psychotherapy, understood as being "designed to transform "false" or "inauthentic" selves into "real" and "authentic" ones (Smith 2005).

Judgments concerning the third, "spirit-relational," form of authenticity involve

(1) one performance (e.g., a shamanistic healing ceremony or a lament) and its effects, which are understood as signs of an interaction between the human performer and an entity whose capacities to bless/heal or curse are understood to exceed merely human capacities;

(2) a second, similar performance and its (e.g., healing) effects, understood similarly to reflect engagement with a more-than-human entity; and

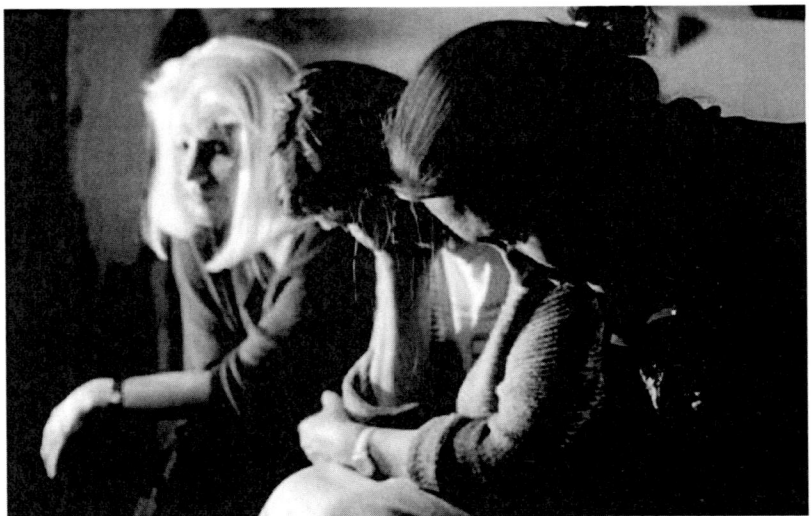

*Figure 3: Still from the Finnish lament documentary* Huomisen Muistoja (Tomorrow's Memories) *by Iiris Härmä (2004).*

(3) a judgment as to the success of performance (2) vis-à-vis (1), and of the likelihood that that success reflects the power in relationship of the performer vis-à-vis the same sort of spirit agency responsible for, say, healing in step (1).

Authentication of a performance as culturally faithful—i.e., authentic in the first sense—entails a metasemiotic judgment about its traditional bona fides. The third type of authentication judgment involves a similar kind of temporality; it compares two temporally separate performances. However, where the first judges the means of performance, the third judges its effects. By contrast with both the cultural and the spirit-relational ver¬sions of authenticity, personal authenticity requires ostensibly rejecting culture as a set of shackles on the true self, and apotheosizes the inner, real, genuine emotional self (Trilling 1972). Its nature as a cultural con¬cept is, paradoxically, to celebrate the self and pretend that its roots and survival do not lie in society or culture. Thus, lamenters who gather with others in a weekend course experience the very sociality they think they have escaped by expressing the pure self and thus (apparently) breaking the chains of culture. To top off these paradoxes, revival leaders—in an echo of Durkheim—regard this achievement cf (a "new") sociality as a process of sacralization.

## Metasemiotic Reflections on Lamenting, Authenticity and the Sacred: Commentary and Judgments vis-à-vis "Traditional" Karelian Lament

*Example 1: Culture-Replicational Authenticity*

During an interview I conducted in 2008 with the most traditionalizing voice in the lament revival, she produced an indirect criticism of ÄI-Lamenters. The critique focused on cultural authenticity (that which is achieved, in this case, through close reproduction of the semiotic forms of traditional laments).

I have found a method that teaches students how to make a lament language that really sounds like [the traditional] lament language although it isn't Karelian. It should be something different from the spoken language [*arkikieli*, the "everyday" Finnish register]. You have to say it in a metaphorical language.

From my later experience as a student in a course this interviewee taught, it became obvious that she advocates not just any metaphors, but the direct translation of the 1,400 canonical metaphors into Finnish.

*Example 2: Spirit-Relational Authenticity: Authentic Power*

Be it for a wedding or a funeral, Karelian villagers evaluated local lamenters in terms of the aftereffects of their laments. Did the marriages she had sanctified with her laments last? Did families remain free of any signs that an unsatisfied dead soul was still close at hand, causing trouble? These questions go to the issue of the spirit-relational authenticity of traditional laments. Even today, the particular confluence of the sacred, the transformative–curative and the psychological in any given lament is closely correlated with that lament's authenticity. "As proof of the lamenter's power was the testimony that 'the master (lamenter) was really good. She gave away 44 girls in marriage and not one was divorced'" (Konkka 1985:107, as cited in Tolbert 1990:47).

*Example 3: Contemporary Lamenters Commenting on Lament's Personal Authenticity*

Having taken pains to lay the foundation for understanding Finnish discourse regarding neolamenting in particular, it is finally time to examine concrete instances of that metasemiotic activity. The discourse transcribed below qualifies as metasemiotic insofar as it involves one act of sign-making, *viz.*, a comment in the semiotic modality of language that objectifies, evaluates and regiments another complex act—lamenting, which involves multiple modes of communication, including weeping, swaying or rocking, voice qualities like the "cry-break" that imitate "normal" crying, and linguistic features.

*Example 4: ÄI-Lamenters' 2009 Annual Meeting*

In the example below, the speaker is Pirkko Fihlman, founder and President of the ÄI-Lamenters. The setting was the Helsinki "Karelia Building" during the ÄI-Lamenters' March 2009 Annual Meeting, which was open to the public. Exceptional publicity—an article in Finland's most prestigious newspaper appearing on the morning of the meeting—led to good attendance (roughly 60 people crowded into a smallish room along with a group of ten invited speakers and ÄI board members.) Following brief presentations by five speakers, the meeting was given over to discussion of lament. Discussion participants were the speakers, board members sitting in the audience and other members of the audience.

Fihlman describes the breakthrough required to actually lament in front of others in ÄI-Lament courses.

It's a **threshold** [*kynnys*] for many. But when one **dares** to go [over the threshold], then that authenticity comes to the fore.

[About 20 seconds skipped]

[We have] the feeling **like being sisters** [*niinku oltas sisaria*]. When we have **authentically** [*aidosti*] faced each other it's that kind of **eternal** [*ikuinen*] friendship that will last and it's fantastic in these days.

Several features of Fihlman's discourse are noteworthy. Fihlman repeatedly invokes (personal-expressive) "authenticity." Note the words in boldface that co-occur with, and reinforce, Fihlman's discourse on "authenticity." They clarify her meaning via metaphors—the threshold, nakedness—and terms (daring, eternal sisterhood) that evoke desirable states. Threshold, nakedness and daring underscore the risk inherent in personal-expressive authenticity, and all are connected to lamenters' invocation of the sacred, and particularly the sacred as dangerous.[7]

A threshold lies between safety and danger in both a spiritual and a psycho-emotional sense (Laurinkienė 2011:57). The threshold of which Fihlman speaks is the decision to express deep and previously unexpressed feelings, which is a frightening prospect (perhaps particularly to Finns [Ådahl 2007:171]).

Nakedness also poses a threat. This theme appears in three expressions, two of which we encounter in later examples:

(1) in Fihlman's discourse, being "without skin" (*nahaton*, i.e., *nahkaton*);

(2) in Tuomas Rounakari's discourse, "nakedness" (*alastamuus*); and

(3) in "Maggie's" discourse, being "undressed" or "stripped" (*riisutusti*).

An act with inherent risk—again, of either a spiritual or a socio-emotional sort—requires "daring" (*uskallus*, from the verb *uskaltaa*). The potential reward for "daring" to cross the "threshold" and share profound feelings in a lament course is the achievement of sisterhood. The term already has a spiritual ring to it, especially in the context of New Age relational spirituality, but its co-occurrence with eternal strengthens the interpretation that the risks and rewards of which Fihlman speaks reflect a sacredness built on the achievement of an I-Thou relationship in the "therapeutic" context of lamenting together.

Let us see how these themes arise in the speech of others involved in lamenting.

*Example 5: Tuomas' Reflection on Authenticity (Nakedness) as Sacred*

The following example represents the way Tuomas Rounakari, Vice-President of ÄI-Lamenters and typically Pirkko's co-teacher in lament courses, links authenticity with sacredness. The fact that he had just been

---

[7] The ambiguity of the sacred is well known. For a specifically Finnish context involving the ambiguity of the sacred, see Koski (2008).

talking about some risks entailed in labeling lament "sacred" helps to explain his emphatic stress on the verb in the final line, "*is,*" marked by capitalization and bolding.

And in the same way, in lament there is that kind of state of spiritual nakedness that *is* sacred in this way.

To paraphrase what Tuomas had just been saying, together with the translated words above: Yes, there are risks in representing lament as sacred—but it *is*! Here, "nakedness" is a metaphorical substitute for "self-revelatory authenticity."

*Example 6: Aino and Pirkko's Dialogue about Depth and Sacredness*

The previous transcripts represent the discourse of ÄI leaders, but current and former participants in ÄI-Lament courses also speak of the importance of authenticity, using some of the same metaphors as Pirkko and Tuomas. The next example involves Pirkko in dialogue with a former student, Aino. Below that I present a striking invocation of authenticity by another student, "Maggie." Just as Aino's words about authenticity and the sacred emerged in dialogue with Pirkko, those same topics were addressed by "Maggie" in Example 7 in a way that built on previous contributions to a multi-party discussion which space does not allow me to include.

The first speaker in Example 6 is Pirkko Fihlman. She begins by affirming the otherness, and hence implicitly the sacredness, of lament. Ignoring for a time the question of what lamenters themselves experience, she then affirms that laments touch others' deepest feelings.

Pirkko: "Laments are not like things in every other sort of place but, they are areas where the deepest feelings that a person had are touched. And then lament should always start with … a prayer."

Aino: "Like I said in the beginning, it's such a sacred thing."

Fihlman begins by indirectly stating that lamenting consists of authentic self-expression—that is, expression of one's deepest feelings—then stating that laments should start with prayer. This defies the outsider's perception that group lamenting is a completely secular activity, serving a psychotherapeutic purpose. Aino responds to Fihlman's indirect statement of lament's sacredness by explicitly asserting it. Quite paradoxically from a perspective that ignores the penetration of psy-discourse by post-secular spirituality, the sacredness of lament for Aino reflects the fact that lamenting involves a semi-public sharing of people's deepest feelings. That is, personal-expressive authenticity is not only required for therapeutic reasons, but for the achievement of "inner life spirituality," in which "mind-body-emotions holism is not strictly secular. And neither is the true, inner self of more humanistic renderings of the ethic of authenticity" (Heelas 2008:175). Psy- is here shown to be undergoing colonization by discourses on spirituality and sacrality.

The trope or metaphor of depth is closely associated with the authentic or true self, a notion of experience that recent centuries of European thought have produced and apotheosized. The trope of depth is not derived naturally. Instead, "a set of phrasings of depth, interiority, and authenticity; sensibilities of holism and transcendence; and practices of reading and writing have crafted a mode of being that many in the West would call experience" (Desjarlais 1994:889). The metaphor of depth is a defining feature of psychoanalytic thought (Wachtel 2003), but also of "inner life spiritualities" in the New Age (Houtman and Aupers 2007; Heelas 2008; Wilce 2011).

*Example 7: A Student's Reflections Following a 2009 Lament Course*

What follows is an excerpt from an interview with "Maggie," who had recently participated in a lament course.

But everyone [usually], you know, tries to give as beautiful as possible and as clever as possible a picture of themselves. And here [by contrast] when one is quite naked with one's feelings, then one is not that beautiful or that clever.

The "here" (*tässä*) that Maggie uttered—defined as that time and place in which one is emotionally "naked, undressed" (*riisutusti*)—is the lament course in which she had participated. Why does she speak of being naked? It may actually be a quotation of her teachers' discourse. She would probably have heard Fihlman or Rounakari invoke nakedness as a metaphor of the kind of emotional revelation that heals by connecting one to oneself and to others in the course.

## Examples 8 and 9: What Sort of "Psychotherapy" Do These Courses Represent?

The following section focuses on jargon used by ÄI-Lamenters that derives from psychodynamic and particularly Freudian therapy. Certain tropes—unconsciousness, psychic defences, et cetera—pervade psychoanalytic discourse and its popular echoes. Lament teachers like Pirkko Fihlman refer to an inner depth of the self as the disturbed, dis-eased burial place of the most recalcitrant feelings, traumas and problems to be dealt with in the context of a healing/therapeutic lament course. In such a course in 2009, Fihlman (Example 8) invokes the *alitajunta* (beneath awareness, subconscious) as she was speaking of

how healing this lamenting is. I was able to get rid of those sorts of things that I never have become 'aware/conscious' [*tiedostanut*] of [...]. In our lament courses [...] one dares [*uskaltaa*] to face those feelings that have stayed unconscious [*alitajunta*].

Lamenters also make indirect reference to repression ("damming up") and catharsis, as when Pirkko spoke the following words during the same course (Example 9):

and when I made that lament I realized how healing lament is, because the kinds of things that I had dammed up [*patoutumia*], came out.

One young course alumna ("Minni") had become exceptionally familiar with the psychological self-help literature and its indirect Freudian roots. Minni referred to defense mechanisms in our April 2009 interview. She embraced the lament course on a number of levels, affirming that the course was aptly named (*Hoitava Itku*, "Healing Lament"), that the traditions of people from eastern Finland (as opposed to her home in the west) had much to contribute to Finland, and that the *itkuprossessi* (lament [course] process)[8] in many ways mimics the ideal process followed by psychodynamically oriented therapists. Yet, Minni argues (somewhat paradoxically) that the indirect, metaphoric expression of feelings in la-

---

[8] For online discourse (in Finnish) concerning the "lament process" posted by *ÄI-Lamenters*, see www.itkuvirsi.net/itkeminen.html.

ment may be more therapeutically efficacious than the direct language advocated in assertiveness training and some forms of psychotherapy.

*Example 10, "Minni": Paradoxes of puolustusmekanismejä (Defense Mechanisms)*

That painful matter can be handled a lot better when using those metaphors. Through this the defense mechanism will break[9]—can break and it breaks more easily when word–images are used, not in that raw way of [speaking about] things.

To this graduate of a lament course, direct ("raw") speech style encouraged in psychotherapy only reinforces distancing, intellectualization or *puolustusmekanismejä* (defense mechanisms). For her, "linguistic images" promote catharsis. In a paradoxical way this imagistic, indirect and "soft" traditional language both covers and reveals. Its indirectness draws a curtain over the act of communication entailed in the lament. Yet even so, Minni argues, the act is achieved.

## Conclusion

The Finnish lament "revival" and its chief manifestation and driver, lament courses, do share features in common with other New Age healing courses. Among others, this includes the lack of any commitment to solely pursue one healing practice. Yet to a unique extent, Finnish lament courses combine the local and global, a particular cultural tradition once rich with sacred overtones and a globally circulating and apparently secular science, namely psy-. In the process they produce a fascinating hybrid. For lamenting in its new context, according to course instructors, is both therapeutic and sacred.

A potential weakness, especially in my model of conceptually distinct authenticities, is: I have associated emotional expression with "personal authenticity," but a powerful emotionality characterized traditional Karelian lamenting as well as the laments encouraged by both the "traditionalist" and the "liberal" wings of the Finnish lament revival. The traditional

---

[9] The mood of the verb *murtenee* is *potential*, indicating likelihood or possibility.

authenticating metadiscourse surrounding old Karelian lamenting represented the lamenter's strong feelings as a sign of her trance possession-like state (Tolbert 1990) in which she communicated with spirits. Contemporary lament practice is an extremely complex cultural (and metacultural, Urban 2001) phenomenon. Depending on which revival leader you speak with, any or all three potential paths of authentication apply to neolament performances. There are literalists who argue that contemporary lament must draw exclusively from the 1,400 (translated) circumlocutions in order to be (culturally) authentic. With apparent exclusivity, other lament leaders aim for the kind of authenticity whose substance is personal self-expression. Spirit-relational authenticity is the rarest of the three authenticities vis-à-vis contemporary lament courses. Yet in private or public, culture replicators and self-revealers admit to having opened the door, by proper lamenting, to relationships with other-than-human beings. If these three paths to authenticity were truly divergent, they would lead to different forms of sacredness. In fact, however, neolamenters may argue that the spirits require use of the "lament language," that they have personally experienced spiritual connections perhaps due to their use of that register, while they also agree that what outsiders looking in on lament courses may see as a completely secular kind of group therapy is to them (as it is to others engaged in post-secular spiritual practices) something sacred. The sacredness of old Karelian laments relies on their use of the language of the spirits. Sacredness for neolamenters requires the creation of an emotionally transparent, person-to-person, I-Thou relationship in a small group. Yet to some extent, allegiance among contemporary lamenters to either a cultural or a personal authenticity continues to divide "traditionalists" and "liberals." Finnish "neolamenters" may in fact feel torn as they try to achieve all three forms of authenticity, that is, as they try to preserve honest personal expressivity while embracing some of the more "restricting" semiotic features of traditional lament, e.g., alliteration and the strict canon of circumlocutions, and privately experience the supernatural in connection with having lamented, apparently both "properly" and (in the third magical–spiritual sense of authenticity) efficaciously.

Earlier in this essay I asserted that concepts of authenticity hold the keys to understanding precisely how the themes of religion, healing, and psychiatry come together in the practice of lamenting in Karelia and Finland. Authenticity once likely denoted the expert lamenter's power whose source is in her fluency in the language of the spirits, her shaman-like acquaintance with those spirits, and her ability to withstand the dangers inherent in lamenting as spiritual work (Tolbert 1990). In revivalist lament courses *aitous* (authenticity) denotes the neolamenter's willingness to "strip" herself in order to reveal her deepest feelings, heal herself, and in the process heal her audience. In either case, authenticity leads to ritual efficacy.

In creating the sacred/healing space that they do—attributing sacredness to the intimacy that emerges in lament courses—ÄI-Lamenters are inventing one among many newly emergent post-secular soteriologies. For ÄI-Lament leaders, the healing quality of group lamenting is not *a value*, but somehow connected to what is now, in the Age of Authenticity, *the ultimate value*. Authenticity-in-facing-the-Other-in-"nakedness" but also in metaphoric expression—i.e., "covered" (poetically mediated) self-exposure—is sacred. And ÄI-Lamenters' mission to heal Finns' "emotional disability" is soteriological; the salvation of Finnish society rests on the success of ÄI's mission. Thus, here in this thoroughly anthropological essay about Finnish lamenting, I have pointed to new combinations of the sacred, the therapeutic and the psychological—new ways of understanding the self, healing and religion—whose relatively unique features may, in fact, be on the verge of spreading through other countries with local traditions waiting to be re-contextualized and put to service in our postmodern world.

**Acknowledgements**

This material is based upon work supported by the National Science Foundation under Grant No. 0822512. Any opinions, findings and conclusions or recommendations expressed in this material are those of the author and do not necessarily reflect the views of the National Science Foundation.

Many thanks to George Gumerman IV and Robert Trotter at Northern Arizona University; to Pertti Anttonen, Heidi Haapoja, Eila Stepanova, Elli-Noora Virkkunen, Pinja Haukkavaara, Lotte Tarkka and the Department of Folkloristics at Helsinki University. My heartfelt gratitude goes to all those in Finland who gave generously of their time, advice, instruction, correction, et cetera, and who allowed me to record and analyze their rich and beautiful discourse.

## References

Ådahl, S. 2007 Good Lives, Hidden Miseries: An Ethnography of Uncertainty in a Finnish Village. Dissertation, Department of Sociology, Helsinki University, Helsinki. www.ethesis.helsinki.fi/julkaisut/val/sosio/vk/adahl/

Agha, A. 2007 Language and Social Relations. Cambridge: Cambridge University Press.

Bruner, E. 1994 Abraham Lincoln as Authentic Reproduction: A Critique of Postmodernism. American Anthropologist 96(2):397–415.

Deleuze, G. 1983 Plato and the Simulacrum. October 27(1):45–56.

Desjarlais, R. R. 1994 Struggling Along: The Possibilities for Experience Among the Homeless Mentally Ill. American Anthropologist 96(4):886–901.

Hanks, W. F. 1996 Language and Communicative Practices. Boulder: Westview.

Heelas, P. 1981 Introduction. *In* Indigenous Psychologies: The Anthropology of the Self. P. Heelas and A. Lock, eds. Pp. 3–18. New York: Academic Press.

———. 2008 Spiritualities of Life: New Age Romanticism and Consumptive Capitalism. Malden, MA: Wiley-Blackwell.

Holloman, R. 1974 Ritual Opening and Individual Transformation: Rites of Passage at Esalen. American Anthropologist 76(2):265–280.

Honko, L. 1963 Itkuvirsirunous. [Lament Poetry] *In* Kirjoittamaton kirjallisuus: Suomen Kirjallisuus [Unwritten Literature: Finnish Literature]. M. Kuusi, ed. Pp. 82–96. Helsinki: Suomalaisen Kirjallisuuden Seura.

Houtman, D., and S. Aupers 2007 The Spiritual Turn and the Decline of Tradition: The Spread of Post-Christian Spirituality in 14 Western Countries, 1981–2000. Journal for the Scientific Study of Religion 46(3):305–320.

Keane, W. 2007 Christian Moderns: Freedom and Fetish in the Mission Encounter. Berkeley: University of California Press.

Kivivuori, J. 1991 Psykokulttuuri: Sosiologinen Näkökulma Arjen Psykologisoitumisen Prosessiin. [Psychoculture: A Sociological Viewpoint to the Psychologisation of Everyday Life] Tampere: Hanki ja jää.

Konkka, U. 1985 Ikuinen Ikävä: Karjalaiset Riitti-Itkut. [Eternal Longing: Karelian Ritual Laments]. Helsinki: Suomalaisen Kirjallisuuden Seura.

Koski, K. 2008 Conceptual Analysis and Variation in Belief Tradition: A Case of Death-Related Beings. Folklore: Electronic Journal of Folklore 38(1):45–56.

Lau, R. W. K. 2010 Revisiting Authenticity: A Social Realist Approach. Annals of Tourism Research 37(2):478–498.

Laurinkiené, N. 2011 Stones-Goddesses in Granaries. Archaeologia Baltica 15:56–60.

Lindholm, C. 2008 Culture and Authenticity. Malden, MA: Blackwell Publishers.

Reddy, W. M. 2001 The Navigation of Feeling: A Framework for the History of Emotions. Cambridge: Cambridge University Press.

Roberts, S. R. 2004 Toasting Uyghurstan: Negotiating Stateless Nationalism in Transnational Ritual Space. Journal of Ritual Studies 18(2):86–105.

Rose, N. 1996 Inventing Our Selves: Psychology, Power, and Personhood. Cambridge: Cambridge University Press.

Smith, B. 2005 Ideologies of the Speaking Subject in the Psychotherapeutic Theory and Practice of Carl Rogers. Journal of Linguistic Anthropology 15(2):258–272.

———. in press The Semiotics and Politics of 'Real Selfhood' in the American Therapeutic Discourse of the World War II Era. Semiotica 203(1/4).

Stepanova, E. 2011 Reflections of Belief Systems in Karelian and Lithuanian Laments: Shared Systems of Traditional Referentiality? Archaeologia Baltica 15:120–143.

Taylor, C. 2007 The Age of Authenticity. *In* A Secular Age. Pp. 473–504. Cambridge: Harvard University Press.

Tolbert, E. 1990 Magico-Religious Power and Gender in the Karelian Lament. *In* Music, Gender, and Culture. M. Herndon and S. Zigler, ed. Pp. 41–56. Wilhelmshaven: Florian Noetzel Verlag.

Trilling, L. 1972 Sincerity and Authenticity. Cambridge: Harvard University Press.

Urban, G. 2001 Metaculture: How Culture Moves through the World. Minneapolis: University of Minnesota Press.

Utriainen, T., T. Hovi, and M. Broo 2012 Combining Choice and Destiny: Identity and Agency within Post-Secular Well-Being Practices. *In* Post-Secular Society. P. Nynäs, M. Lassander, and T. Utriainen, eds. Pp. 187–216. New Brunswick, NJ: Transaction Publishers.

Wachtel, P. L. 2003 The Surface and the Depths: The Metaphor of Depth in Psychoanalysis and the Ways in which it can Mislead. Contemporary Psychoanalysis 39(1):5–26.

Wang, N. 1999 Rethinking Authenticity in Tourism Experience. Annals of Tourism Research 26(2):349–370.

Wilce, J. M. 2009 Language and Emotion. Cambridge: Cambridge University Press.

———. 2011 Sacred Psychotherapy in the Age of Authenticity: Healing and Cultural Revivalisms in Contemporary Finland. Religions 2(4):566–589.

## Chapter 12

## Healing Enchantment: How Does Angel-Healing Work?

*Terhi Utriainen*

**Introduction**

What we call "alternative therapies" are once again challenging secular therapies. We may thus ask if we are, partly, stepping into a post-secular culture of healing, or if, on the contrary, we ever were very secular in terms of our aspirations and methods of healing after all (Nynäs, Lassander and Utriainen 2012; cf. Latour 1993, 2010; Orsi 2005). Many people in the West today combine therapies with different backgrounds or prefer non-official and not completely secular methods to alleviate at least some forms of their malaise.[1] Alternative or complementary healing takes many forms, one branch of them being energy-healing with its different sub-categories (Utriainen, Hovi and Broo 2012:194).[2] In this chapter my focus will be on one relative newcomer in the Western field of energy-healing, namely, angel-healing as it was present in my ethnographic multi-method study in Finland. I ask: Why do angels appear as contemporary healing aids and figures? What are today's healing angels like and how do people turn to them? What exactly happens in angel-therapy and how could we approach its claim of efficacy—or its magic? I propose as at least a partial answer that angels provide healing enchantment and highlight hybrid or participatory agency.

---

[1] See Verrips (2003) for how the popular imagination not only sees medical doctors as secular scientists but also as magicians that both create and destroy life. The complex question "how magic belongs to modernity" is addressed from various angles in Meyer and Pels (2003).

[2] The classic study on ritual healing in Western society is McGuire (1989); see also Bowmann (1999, 2000), Hovi (2012), Pohjanheimo (2012), McPherson (2008) and Wood (2000). On well-being and healing practices in post-secular society, see Utriainen, Hovi and Broo (2012).

My research project focuses on contemporary practices with angels and the everyday lives that host these practices.[3] The material on which my reflections are based comes basically from four groups of sources: (1) interviews with approximately 20 Finnish people who work and communicate with angels; (2) participatory observation during an angel-therapy training course and several other angel-related settings; (3) a questionnaire (N 263) distributed at the lecture by the Irish writer and angel-seer Lorna Byrne[4] in Helsinki and (4) diverse media material, literature and other cultural artifacts. Angel spirituality in general and its healing aspects in particular have become increasingly popular in Finland during the last five to ten years. This phenomena has, for instance, received media attention in women's magazines and tabloids, talk shows and, occasionally, also in the news media (Utriainen 2013b). The Evangelical Lutheran Church of Finland has also developed an interest in this growing phenomenon, which attracts many church members.[5] Recently, the popularity of angels has also been studied, for instance, in the US, UK, Germany, Norway, Hungary and Estonia (Draper and Barker 2010; Gardella 2007; Walter 2011, 2016; Murken 2009; Gilhus 2012; Kis-Halas 2012; Uibu 2013). Thus we are dealing with a phenomenon not restricted to Finland but that might be called a vivid aspect of contemporary Western folk or vernacular religion (Draper and Barker 2010; Walter 2016).

All the abovementioned studies note that one feature of the present-day popularity of angels is the combination of Christian and esoteric spirituality. For example, in a focus group interview, three women who identified themselves as Lutheran stated that if it was not for angels, they might not have been drawn to alternative spirituality in the first place. What is new in these practices is thus not so much the figure of an angel in itself (be-

---

[3] This research is part of the larger project "Post-secular culture and a changing religious landscape in Finland" being conducted at Åbo Akademi University 2010–2014.
[4] Lorna Byrne has become increasingly popular worldwide and also in Finland, where her two autobiographical books, *Angels in my Hair* (2008) and *Stairway to Heaven* (2010), have sold extremely well. She has visited Finland three times. See www.lornabyrne.com.
[5] According to the Church Monitor 2007, 46.1 percent of Finns believe in angels; on the growing interest in angels see Kirkon Tutkimuskeskus (2012:40).

ing part of Christian imaginary and chain of memory) but some of the (sometimes "magical") ways in which angels are communicated with. Attraction to angels and angel-healing can thus be taken as at least a weak signal or indication of what contemporary women in Western societies might desire from healing and therapeutic religion (Utriainen 2014).

In the Christian tradition angels are messengers of God occupying a space between the divine and the human. Sometimes these messengers appear in human form, but they can also take other visual and sensitive appearances—they can, for instance, appear as figures of light. Since in Christian and especially in Lutheran theology angels are relatively loosely defined figures, they can easily be transferred to many kinds of more or less vaguely defined spiritual settings, such as New Age.[6] In art and popular parlance, angels often work as metaphors of God's mercy, beauty, inspiration and goodness. Today angels have become a vivid figure and element of volatile modern lives, as much in entertainment and commerce as in healing.[7] The French philosopher Michel Serres in his book *La Légende des Anges* uses the figure of an angel to exemplify the overall volatile nature of present-day life.

Traditionally, active angels have appeared to relatively passive humans as receivers of godly grace or punishment—in one word, as powerful. This has been the case in traditional miracle stories reporting angelic interventions, especially in the contexts of accidents, acute illnesses, on a person's deathbed or in visions of the apocalypse where angels carry God's fury.[8] We can also find the active angel and the relatively passive woman in the famous motif of the annunciation: the archangel Gabriel delivers the message of the birth of the son of God to the young girl Mary, who either humbly or slightly resentfully accepts the reported miracle. By contrast, today people seem to take a much more active role in their encounters with angels than Mary has been depicted as doing. Instead of

---

[6] In fact, according to Ingvild Gilhus (2012), in Norway angels have become intriguing and disturbing border markers between state Lutheranism and New Age. Something similar could be said concerning Finland.

[7] See Draper and Baker (2010) and Gardella (2007) for an overview of North American angel culture. For angels as one effective power in one traditional Hungarian healer's repertoire, see Kis-Halas (2012).

[8] About fierce angels in the US evangelical imagination, see Gardella (2007:168–199).

waiting for God to send angels to them, they reach for angels, summon angels and ask them to act with them toward several ends. There are various, overlapping methods for reaching out to angels, such as oracle cards, meditations, talismans and healing.

My research participants—most of them women[9]—report taking angels into their lives to better cope, stay healthy and creative and enjoy or merely support their lives. Their angelic world is a creative collage of biblical, apocryphal, theosophical and New Age elements; these traditions are emphasized differently in the different accounts. The most important categories of angels for them are archangels and personal (guardian) angels—the latter are the best known angelic figures in traditional Lutheran culture. All archangels have their own attributes, particular fields of action and energy, weekdays and colors. For instance, Michael's color is deep blue and his energy is protective, whereas Gabriel's color is white and he is responsible for guidance and insight.[10] Personal (guardian) angels are more idiosyncratic and often in very intimate and reciprocal relations with humans. When needed, they can help connect humans with more powerful angels in the angelic hierarchy. Angels can be understood either as coming from the personal Christian God or from some much more general and abstract source of universal life. It is thus possible to say that the present-day religiosity/spirituality[11] around angels combines theistic and holistic tones and aspirations and this combination may be one factor that makes angels a popular and effective source of healing in today's world and particularly in societies with a strong Christian heritage.

---

[9] According to my survey, 94 percent of those who came to listen to Lorna Byrne in Helsinki were women. On the predominance of women in many forms of religion, as well as the sociological explanations given to this phenomenon, see Trzebiatowska and Bruce (2012). For the history and change of women's religion in Finland, see Utriainen and Salmesvuori (2014).

[10] Raphael is often depicted as a green or turquoise healing power; Uriel is purple and his field is forgiveness; Jofiel is yellow and joyful and Samuel is pink and represents and embodies love.

[11] See Utriainen, Hovi, and Broo (2012) for our reasons for using the slash. It basically means that the distinction between religion and spirituality should be taken as an emic rather than etic one.

## Emotions and Depression

Some of my research participants are semiprofessional practitioners of angel-therapy and other forms of healing, but many are laypersons who started their "spiritual path" some years earlier. They come mostly from lower and mid-middle classes and have a variety of educational backgrounds: of those who took part in our survey, one-fourth work in commerce and administration, many in teaching and the health and social sectors. Nearly one-fifth has a university degree. The majority (73.8 percent) belongs to the Lutheran Church of Finland,[12] even though only a very few consider themselves active members. The most important thing about the Church for interviewees is its important social work, and they identify themselves as "spiritual individuals" who find their own spirituality mostly outside the Church. Some are also active yoga practitioners, and many have practiced Reiki or other forms of holistic or energy-healing.[13] Since the vast majority of research participants were women, I will focus on them.[14] Let us first consider the women's reasons for turning to angels. These reasons reveal not only "holistic" distress, but also the fact that depression is not an uncommon experience in today's life.

The survey (N 263) indicates why women turn to angels and other spiritual practices: to find aid and support in various distressing experiences in life like depression and illness; to seek spiritual growth, development, guidance and better knowledge of oneself and one's emotions; to support their faith and confidence; to be healed; to release stress; for general well-being and clarity of thought and of one's life and to find energy, joy and a connection and support for one's choices. Apart from "faith" and "spir-

---

[12] The overall rate in Finland in 2011 is 77.2 percent.
[13] The range of healing activities was pretty much similar to that encountered by Wood (2000:83) during his ethnographic research in Nottinghamshire. See also Bowman (1999).
[14] In the survey there were 248 women and 15 men. Of the 24 interviewees 19 were women. All the women interviewed live or have lived in heterosexual relations, most of them have children, and their ages range from 30 to 70 years. They include a nurse, a yoga teacher, a sales assistant, a singer, a stylist, an artist, and a congregation worker. The men interviewed were a husband to an angel-healer, two friends who had a long history in theosophy as well as two young yoga practitioners who had taken part in an angel meditation week at their yoga school.

itual growth," an explicitly religious and particularly Christian vocabulary of sin, guilt, remorse and forgiveness is absent—even though well over 70 percent are members of the Lutheran Church of Finland.

The interviews provide long and often detailed autobiographical accounts of the various ups and downs in their lives. Nearly all the accounts include a period of crises, like illnesses, unemployment and very often clinically diagnosed depression. Many report finding clarity and relief in their own often complex and confused emotional life through angels—so much so that working with angels could, to a large extent, be said to be about emotion work and improvement of self-knowledge (cf. Riis and Woodhead 2010; Utriainen 2014; see also Uibu 2013; Walter 2014).

> Four or three . . . years ago I suffered from severe depression and was taken to the hospital. It was in fact very soon after that, that I painted these angels . . . Maybe I got to know myself a little better.
>
> Very, very big challenges, yes, yes. So that perhaps without Reiki and the help of angels I wouldn't ever have been able to bear it. But they gave me some extra strength so that in a way I felt that I always went from one stage to another . . . I have been in very heavy moods and heavy phases of life. I have all the time gone forward, it becomes easier and lighter.

As expressed in the above quotes, the interviewees relate how they use angels to find their way out of difficult and heavy phases of life, to learn to improve self-knowledge and knowledge of their emotions and to obtain a stronger sense that they can make a difference and become agents of their own lives. However, one important feature of these stories of empowerment and healing is the emphasis on not needing to be alone— not needing to carry complex everyday responsibilities without support: angels act as companions and partners in practically all spheres and moments of life (from very practical needs such as finding parking places and lost objects to more spiritual aspirations like protecting one's children and finding one's path and purpose). One of my informants summarizes her experience accordingly: "I do everything with them. It is not like I wouldn't have angels and God present: they are here all the time."

The survey data also includes the response of one crisis therapist. She reports that she decided to go and listen to the Irish angel-seer Lorna Byrne's lecture on angels precisely because she increasingly meets patients who seek help from angel-related and other spiritual practices and wanted to see for herself what it was about; in the questionnaire she states that she was impressed by the "strength of faith" she was able to witness at the event. This individual piece of information indicates that there are interesting and complex negotiations between the spiritual and secular therapeutic fields.[15] If we combine this with insights from the survey and interviews, both angel-healers and their "clients"[16] emphasize that angel-healing, along with other kinds of alternative healing, is often both more subtle and effective than either the churchly pastoral care or the secular social and therapeutic services that are provided today. But what is the economic cost of angel-healing? One of my interviewees reflects on money in the following terms, explaining how the best teachers and healers are often not the most expensive ones:

Well, I could have some other hobbies that would take the same amount of money, and it is pretty expensive also to go to yoga or aerobic . . . For the sake of the children, I can't take many courses a year. And I try to choose teachers who are authentic [who don't charge too much].[17]

## What Happens in Angel-Healing?

Scholars such as Gillian Bennett and Robert Orsi have emphasized how modern history has systematically over centuries worked toward downplaying the credibility of the belief in the presence of the supernatural (Bennett 1987; Orsi 2005). Read against this background, it is interesting that many of the interviewees voice their joy of an "increasing" tolerance in society toward invisible and extraordinary aspects of life. They feel that the presence of the invisible otherworld and the enchanted sentiments it triggers are gaining more public attention, for instance, in the media.

---

[15] In 2008 in Finland there was an attempt to formulate a law restricting alternative and belief-based medicinal practices basically in order to protect vulnerable individuals. While this specific law proposal was dropped, concerns with alternative medicine prevail and attempts to regulate it continue.

[16] The term "client" as opposed to "patient" is preferred by my angel-healer interviewees. This relates to the fact that these therapies are often structured as small entrepreneurial activities.

[17] See Wood's (2000:85) comparison of the price of a holistic healing session and a night out at the pub.

But how is the particular enchantment of angel-healing effectuated and in what ways is it understood as healing? By enchantment I am referring to meaning-making and relational practices and operations engaged with forces or entities that are in some sense believed and used to resource, enrich and support mundane or secular lives. My guideline here comes from Jane Bennett: "To be enchanted is to be struck and shaken by the extraordinary that lives amid the familiar and the everyday" (Bennett 2001:5). Bennett also notes that enchantment is not always a spontaneous happening but can be fostered through deliberate action. Enchantment thus engages the bigger or smaller extraordinary (which could sometimes be called alterity or transcendence) either as a surprise or as something desired, summoned and invited (see also Csordas 2004; Luckmann 1990; Utriainen 2013a). The presence of invisible and extraordinary actors is a constitutive aspect of angel-healing, and the felt effect of the healing ritual is related to how this presence is called for and incorporated. In healing enchantment, the embodiment of the healer becomes a combination, or a hybrid, of human and other-than-human elements and "energies."

What follows is a description of an angel-healing technique in which this kind of enchantment is at play. This description is given from the viewpoint of the healer or, more precisely, the apprentice healer participating in a training course who sometimes also assumes the role of the *healée*.[18] I propose that what takes place is a process of artful and well-structured *enchantment, which somehow becomes healing*. I will in the following draw some comparisons with Tanya Luhrmann's ethnography on modern urban magic as well as with research on other healing techniques.

The angel-healer course was organized during the winter of 2011–12; it was two weekends, and there was more than a month between the weekends, in which individuals were given homework to complete. The course was held in the home of the female teacher-healer in Helsinki. The participants were familiarized with angel traditions (such as the old Christian angel hierarchies) and with some concrete angel-healing techniques. There were six female participants (including me) between the ages of 30 and 55; three lived a distance from the metropolitan area. Three were planning to start a practice of angel-healing and the other three were al-

---

[18] This expression is inspired by Marion Bowman.

# Healing Enchantment

ready engaged in some alternative healing methods which they practiced as entrepreneurs.

We were told about various healing methods, but the following model depicts the one we practiced most both in the role of healer and *healée*. The materials on which my reflections are based are my field notes and the course material given to the students. The most important source is the 60-page workbook written by the teacher and used throughout the course, including for homework; many of my field notes were written on the pages of this book while we studied. It is important to bear in mind that the ethnographic situation was not actual healing but a pedagogical course for healers to be, which means this analysis can be merely heuristic.

*Preparation: The healer lights a candle (and may play some background music). The healer gives the* healée *water and asks her to sit/lie down. The healer brings her hands together and thanks her personal angel and connects with it. The healer puts her hands on the shoulders of the* healée. *The healer asks the personal angel of the* healée *to come along The healer asks the* healée *to move (in her mind) into her own sacred place. The healer also moves into her own sacred place (closes her eyes).*

*Invocation of the Angels: The healer (with her hands together) asks the archangel Michael to come and spread his wings as she spreads her arms around the* healée *(opens her arms); she asks Michael to pour his protective bright blue energy over the* healée. *After some minutes the healer thanks Michael and lets him go (and closes her arms). This invocation (with the opening and closing of hands) is repeated individually for all seven archangels.*

*Closing: The healer thanks all the archangels, including her own and the* healée's *personal angels. She asks the* healée *to leave her sacred place and the healer also leaves her own. She touches the shoulder of the* healée *(and wakes her up). She offers a glass of water. She asks if the* healée *feels okay.*

*Interpretation: The healer asks the* healée *how she felt during the healing. She leads a discussion about the sensations and mental images and their possible meanings.*

Dividing the healing session into four parts is my construction. However, I maintain that these divisions (preparation, invocation, closing and interpretation) could easily be found by any observer. This angel-healing session usually lasts about 30 minutes and most of it, especially the invocation, happens in silence. However, the healer-trainee is taught to observe in detail her own feelings and sensations during the whole session and to be ready to put them into words afterward. The vocabularies formed (words describing and interpreting sensations) are thus given special epistemic value: they are articulated as referring to the presence of healing angelic energies, that is, to something invisible that is present during the healing session in the physical and "energetic" interspace between the healer and the *healée*. The angel-healer should gradually learn, during the course and subsequent practice, to observe and articulate this bodily, emotional and imaginary space during the session as proof of the touch of the invisible reality. (Apart from a light touch on the shoulders in the preparation and closing sections, the healer does not physically touch the *healée*.)

## Therapeutic Sensations

The relatively simple bodily choreography in the invocation (in this case it consists most importantly of the spreading and closing of one's arms in invocation or mimesis of the wings of the angels) connects it to the middle of the healing rite and divides it into something like symmetrical subchapters, each of which is dedicated to one archangel. Any sensation (e.g., the feeling of moving air or pressure in some part of the healer's body) or mental image (such as colorful vibrations or flashes of light) arising in the healer during the session can be interpreted as a special need or tension in the client that needs healing or as the intensified presence and touch of a particular angel.

Also, Tanya Luhrmann emphasizes the importance of disciplined training and repetition when learning to organize and decipher the meaningful feelings and other details in the magical rite:

Magicians report a gamut of emotional, spiritual and physiological responses in ritual, and they attribute these experiences to the presence of power in the rite. Magicians will "feel" the power flowing, "feel" the current run around the circle. They often assert that they know whether rituals raise any power because they can sense power intuitively during the ritual . . . Magical power is also thought to be the sort of thing that requires training to handle properly, and some of the magician's responses are attributed to inadequate training for the experience. [Luhrmann 1989:133]

It is possible that silence and speechlessness (especially during the invocation) provide an important space for the detailed differentiations of sensations and mental images. The subsequent act of interpretation provides time and space for the verbal interpretations of the sensations and mental images of both the healer and *healée*. According to the instructions given to our group, the healer should now ask the *healée* whether she felt something (even the smallest sensation) and whether she wishes to talk about it. If she does, the healer listens and helps her to interpret these sensations in terms of an angelic presence; she also brings up some of her own sensations for *comparison* and *reflection*.

This more or less interactive interpretation—which is however led by the healer—should proceed with care, respecting the client's idiosyncrasies toward angels and the otherworld (e.g., in more or less Christian terms). Throughout the course we were reminded of the most important value that the healer must respect absolutely: the free will of every individual and *healée*. (In angel-culture rhetoric, individual free will is something that angels are also said to always respect. Interestingly, free will is a "sacred" value in both Christianity and modern Enlightenment thinking, albeit in somewhat different ways.)

If the healer receives a very powerful sensation during the session, she sometimes talks about it straight away—or it may even spontaneously come out of her mouth. However, since it is understood that everything in the healing, including the words, only comes through her ("is channeled"), we are told that we might not even remember our words later on. It is emphasized that whatever happens is not really considered to be of our making or responsibility. In any case, the healer learns to interpret both her and her client's nuanced sensations and mentalizations as indices of (the need for) the healing power of an angelic presence or energy.

The articulation of the sensations in order to learn about the inner states in many ways resembles mindfulness, yoga and other forms of body-consciousness practices, in which bodily sensations are "read" as messages of mental states. It is also similar to the traditional skill of fortune-tellers and seers in "reading feelings"—both of the specialist and the client—as omens and premonitions (e.g., Bennett 1987:128). Angel-healing here also resembles, in some respects, other alternative healing settings; for instance, an important element in the homeopath's appointment in Finland is a careful and time-consuming interpretation of bodily and mental symptoms and personality features (Lindfors 2005). Quite intriguingly, the angel-healing technique also bears some resemblances to the psychoanalyst's method of countertransference, where, by reading her own sensations and emotions, the therapist may gain information about the patient and her problems. Thus, by focusing on sensations as knowledge the method of angel-healing comes close to many body-consciousness techniques, and in its intersubjective interpretation of sensations and emotions it is also reminiscent of such mental techniques as clairvoyance as well as psychotherapy—when it mimics or genuinely shares some of the same premises. Hence there seem to be many common elements (the interactive structures of the ritual techniques, manners and sequences) in many different kinds of healings and therapies along the spectrum modern–secular to traditional–enchanted.[19]

The general idea in healing with energy or spirits is that the healer only mediates cosmic/divine energy to the *healée*. In the end angels are also to be understood as only mediators of this healing energy. That is why the healer is advised to keep herself as pure and clear (of pollution such as negative thoughts) as possible—which is a common idea in energy-healing (cf. McPherson 2008). However, the interviewees may also admit that purity is an ideal that is not always totally achieved. One healer writes down messages she receives in her channeling, because she feels that it helps her to distinguish what the authentic message meant for her from the input of her own ego: "I must write [it down] because from that writing you see at once if it is pure text or if something from yourself has gone into it . . . Because I am not yet so skillful that everything could come through all clear."

The clarity and purity of the mind and emotions are also important goals of healing, as emphasized for instance in the published material of

---

[19] Verrips (2003:234) gives as examples of similar practices both the fortune-teller and biomedical doctors, who use "glassy materials . . . to achieve more knowledge and deeper insights," that is, the crystal ball, in the first case, and several kinds of lenses and objects, such as the microscope, in the second. Also the homeopath (Lindfors 2005:86), in a similar manner to traditional medical doctors, consults a thick book to verify diagnoses.

Doreen Virtue, one of the most internationally known angel-therapists, who is also often mentioned by my research participants.[20] The idea is that when the *healée* fully experiences the flow of pure angelic energy coming through the healer, she may learn to become the "channel" for her own healing—and start to heal others too.[21] This also legitimizes the idea that the healer (being merely an empty channel) is not, in the end, responsible or the one to be credited for what happens in the session; the healer is, rather, only one joint or mechanism in the interlinking network of the channels that communicate universal healing energy.

**Healing Enchantment**

If the above described and analyzed angel-healing and other angel-practices (such as meditations, card readings, etc.) are viewed as embodied pedagogical practices, their stated aim would be to teach the *healée* to learn to contact angel-energies whenever needed and to use them to enrich quotidian life. They thus aim, at least partly, to enhance self-help and self-healing practices; hence, the hierarchical structure that often differentiates and distances the roles and positions of the healer and the *healée* is relativized. In fact, some healers in my interviews state that it is not advisable to visit an angel-healer too many times, but that they encourage their clients to find their own ways to heal themselves. This blurring of the boundary between the roles and positions of the healer and the *healée* can be regarded as a characteristic feature within alternative healing culture (cf. Woodhead and Sointu 2008). It is also part of the individualist self-help ethos of late modernity.

This easily learnable and portable skill of enchantment is interpreted and valued as an art of life that protects, nurtures, inspires, guides and empowers—and this may be what healing is all about here. I call this healing

---

[20] See, for example, her *Angel Therapy Meditations* CD (2008). For more about her methods, see www.angeltherapy.com.

[21] Wood (2000) writes about two typical ideal routes to power in healing, the closed and the open route, and notes that for instance in Reiki the therapists move from the closed one (only some people can contact the power) to the open one (power can be contacted by everyone). In angel-healing there seems to be the idea that each person can learn to channel the angelic energy on his or her own.

by enchantment, or healing enchantment, meaning that it seems to be enchantment (subtle magic and spell, the well-managed touch of the invisible and extraordinary) that heals. What is created and constructed in angel-healing by its body–mind technique is a special form of imaginary–practical-embodied enchantment (visualizations, feelings and sensations, as well as gestures and postures of connecting and being with angels). And it is this enchantment, actively and skillfully cultivated contact with the invisible, protective and transformative otherness, and what is done with it, that is deemed and experienced as healing. In a somewhat similar way, Luhrmann reports on the modern practitioners of magic and how they treat everything available in the ritual as effective and as a source of transformation and knowledge:

> In magic, the unconscious is not treated as a random, frightening source of subjectivity. Magicians redefine the apparent randomness of instincts and emotions as a knowledge, a matter of sensing, intuiting, feeling the interconnections of the world. Priestesses gaze into fires and crystal to read the symbols revealed to them there . . . The apparently chaotic irrational does not control us; it itself becomes the means of control, by providing an understanding of the natural world. [Luhrmann 1989:90]

But why is enchantment experienced as healing? One approach might be to elaborate the concepts of the imaginary and fantasy (angels as imaginary others and friends) and their impact on (mental) well-being (see Murken 2009). Another and slightly different elaboration might be Thomas Csordas' phenomenological understanding of alterity (otherness, difference) as a source of many kinds of transformations and dislocations (from what is to what becomes). Following Csordas, alterity is not an (theological) object, but is instead seen as an elementary aspect of the embodied and as a relational open structure of human experience, which is always in a process of transformation and dislocation: our changing bodies, desires and suffering, imagination, other people, orientating toward what is not there in both a big and small[22] or frightening and adventurous sense.

---

[22] Thomas Luckmann (1990) also writes about big and small transcendences—although Csordas does not refer to him.

Alterity is neither objective nor absolute. In the sense in which I am using it, alterity is an elementary constituent of subjectivity and intersubjectivity, and this is how it is part of the structure of being in the world. Not only can it be elaborated into the monstrous as well as the divine but it can be transformed into identity, intimacy, or familiarity. [Csordas 2004:164; see also Utriainen 2013a]

What we call "religions" would also evolve from this more general source or kernel of alterity.

The future (in the sense of time not yet to come but becoming) can also be understood as a temporal aspect of alterity, and so would one's "path" or destiny in life. One of the interviewees highlights how her life with angels' alterity, as the unknown future, transformed from uncertainty to adventure:

And because nothing is permanent, the only permanent thing is change, that's for sure . . . we can't lean on anything, because everything changes all the time and there are new tasks waiting all the time . . . and they [the angels] send me to some unbelievable spots, and that's the funniest thing here that life becomes so extremely exciting.

Here angels become the needed tint of magic transporting the individual from uncertainty to adventure.

Besides the transformation from uncertainty to adventure (which in itself can be considered a great achievement), there are other important transitions that can be aspired to with the help of angels. One is the transition—and the skill of mastering this transition—between metaphor (imagination) and magic (concretely felt efficacy). The use of imagination was strongly encouraged throughout the angel-healer course as a means of invoking angels if and when one did not straightforwardly believe in them—belief was not considered a requirement for successful contact. It thus seems that angels can be understood as symbols or metaphors of various positive values. But in some ritual practices, like healing, their metaphoricity is, at least in the specific context at hand and for a limited time and purpose, transformed into "magical" executive power that changes things in a way that can be understood and felt as healing (Utriainen in press). In this way angels may be a very potent yet subtle and flexible vehicle of continuous transformation, inspiration and hope, as well as, for the practitioner, a source of the sense of being able to actively become a doer and maker of one's life and destiny. However, an individual would not be the sole maker of this transformation.

## Conclusion: Enchanted Agency with Others

It is important to note that angel-healing explicitly highlights alterity and relational or participatory agency: agency (e.g., in decision-making situations) which is not reducible to the self alone but is much more open, relational and elastic. The linguistic anthropologist Laura Ahearn provides a short, open and pragmatic definition of agency as a "socioculturally mediated capacity to act" (Ahearn 2001:118). This implies that agency should be taken as a relational and mediated action. As the communication scholar Karlyn Campbell further reminds us, the individual is only one important point of articulation of agency (Campbell 2005).

Angel-healers (i.e., those who have learned how to heal themselves with angels) are understood as working together with angels. A recurring expression in the interviews was "it was not me/I did not make it happen." Thus, angel-healing enhances the sense of individual agency on the one hand ("I use angels to make things happen in my life"); on the other hand, it seems important to attribute agency not only to the self but also to an open and sustaining relationality that includes other possible powers. Enchanted participatory agency would, thus, provide a potentially valuable tool for living within the constraints and possibilities of modernity—in particular to help persons escape from loneliness and, if we take seriously what Alain Ehrenberg writes in *Fatigue d'Être Soi* (2000), possibly to protect the often very solitary subject from depression, which has become a contemporary curse and which was also frequently mentioned in the interviews.

From this perspective, angels as therapists and intimate others appear more and more as a creative healing help for modern individuals who want to keep their lives and futures in their own hands (and who thus continue to appreciate "free will"), who also welcome support, companionship and "miraculous" interventions. One particular further therapeutic feature of angels is that they (and the spirituality as well as the approach to healing that they represent) are completely nonjudgmental. Amy Schindler discusses the ways in which angels became important for

HIV patients in the US in the 1980s, when institutional religions often judged homosexual behavior negatively (1999). Modern angels don't judge personal failures or weaknesses and they seem to understand the profound complexities of life. Matthew Wood, writing on the basis of his ethnography on energy-healing settings, suggests that in some contemporary spiritual activities "healing is called for in a general way, almost as an element of *sustenance*, rather than as a more acute method to counter a specific prevailing condition" (Wood 2000:84; italics mine). The italics are mine since I want to draw attention to this intriguing idea of *healing as sustenance*, that is, as nourishment, as something that feeds and keeps the subject alive.

Enchanted and agentive relations with others can be felt as empowering and healing in some cases and phases of life. However, in other cases, relations with religious alterity may be felt as painful and disempowering. Alterity—and religion—can go to both ways, and the "power of as if" (if we borrow William James' way of capturing the dynamic, metaphoric nature of religion) is potent but also risky. What I also want to stress, and what my interviews and ethnography make visible, as well as Luhrmann's ethnography of modern urban witches, is that an enchanted and potentially healing and sustaining partnership is created, re-created, scrutinized and maintained in embodied relational practice, and that this includes such things as the active use of the imagination, following rules and committing oneself to exercise and repetition—on an individual basis as well as with many kinds of other persons. This implies that such healing does not happen in just a private world but in many ways a very relational one. Furthermore, the above described practices with angels is circulated and informed, but quite possibly also motivated, by such "secular" processes as the crumbling present state of welfare services in Western societies and the pressing, if ambiguous, ethos of autonomy and individualism that guides people to take responsibility of their own lives. What is also involved and merits more attention than it has received in this article is the growing supply of commercial spiritual culture, with its commodities and methods of enchantment, and how it has become involved in healing practices.

# References

Ahearn, L. 2001 Language and Agency. Annual Review of Anthropology 30:109–137.

Asad, T. 1993 Remarks on the Anthropology of the Body. *In* Religion and the Body. S. Coakley, ed. Pp. 42–51. Cambridge: Cambridge University Press.

Bennett, G. 1987 Traditions of Belief: Women and the Supernatural. Hammondsworth: Penguin.

Bennett, J. 2001 The Enchantment of Modern Life: Attachments, Crossings, and Ethics. Princeton: Princeton University Press.

Bowman, M. 1999 Healing in the Spiritual Marketplace: Consumers, Courses and Credentialism. Social Compass 46(2):181–189.

Bowman, M., ed. 2000 Healing and Religion. Middlesex: Hisarlik Press.

Campbell, K. K. 2005 Agency: Promiscuous and Protean. Communication and Critical/Cultural Studies 2(1):1–19.

Csordas, T. J. 2004 Asymptote of the Ineffable: Embodiment, Alterity and the Theory of Religion. Current Anthropology 45(2):163–185.

Draper, S., and J. Barker 2010 Angelic Belief as American Folk Religion. Sociological Forum 26:623–643.

Ehrenberg, A. 2000 [1998] La fatigue d'être soi: Dépression et société. Paris: O. Jacob.

Gardella, P. 2007 American Angels: Useful Spirits in the Material World. Lawrence, KS: University of Kansas.

Gilhus, I. S. 2012 Angels in Norway: Religious Border-crossers and Border-markers. *In* Vernacular Religion in Everyday Life: Expressions of Belief. M. Bowman and Ü. Valk, eds. Pp. 230–245. Sheffield: Equinox.

Hovi, T. 2012 Clinical Services Instead of Sermons. *In* Post-Secular Religious Practices. T. Ahlbäck, ed. Pp. 128–144. Turku: Donner Institute for Research in Religious and Cultural History.

Kirkon, T., ed. 2012 Haastettu kirkko: Suomen evankelis-luterilainen kirkko vuosina 2008–2011. [The Church Challenged: The Evangelical Lutheran Church of Finland in 2008–2011.] Tampere: Church Research Institute.

Kis-Halas, J. 2012 'I Make My Saints Work': A Hungarian Holy Healer's Identity Reflected in Autobiographical Stories and Folk Narratives. *In* Vernacular Religion in Everyday Life: Expressions of Belief. M. Bowman and Ü. Valk, eds. Pp. 63–92. Sheffield: Equinox.

Latour, B. 1993 We Have Never Been Modern. Cambridge: Harvard University Press.

———. 2010 On the Modern Cult of Factish Gods. Durham, NC: Duke University Press.

Lindfors, P. 2005 Homeopaatin Vastaanotolla [At the Appointment of the Homeopath]. Tampere: Tampere University Press.

Luckmann, T. 1990 Shrinking Transcendence, Expanding Religion? Sociological Analysis 50(2):127–138.

Luhrmann, T. 1989 Persuasions of the Witch's Craft: Ritual Magic and Witchcraft in Present-day England. Cambridge: Harvard University Press.

McGuire, M. 1988 Ritual Healing in Suburban America. New Brunswick: Rutgers University Press.

McPherson, J. 2008 Women and Reiki: Energetic/Holistic Healing in Practice. Sheffield: Equinox.

Meyer, B., and P. Pels, eds. 2003 Magic and Modernity: Interfaces of Revelation and Concealment. Stanford: Stanford University Press.

Murken, S. 2009 Mein Wille geschehe... Religionspsychologische Überlegungen zum Verhältnis von Religion und Wunscherfüllung. Zeitschrift für Religionswissenschaft 17: 165–187.

Nynäs, P., M. Lassander, and T. Utriainen 2012 Post-Secular Society. New Brunswick: Transaction Publishers.

Orsi, R. 2005 Between Heaven and Earth: The Religious Worlds People Make and the Scholars Who Study Them. Princeton: Princeton University Press.

Partridge, C. 2004 The Re-Enchantment of the West. Vol. 1. London: Continuum.

Pohjanheimo, O. 2012 The Enrichment of Magical Thinking through Practices among Reiki Self-Healers. *In* Post-Secular Religious Practices.

T. Ahlbäck, ed. Pp. 289–312. Turku: Donner Institute for Research in Religious and Cultural History.

Riis, O., and L. Woodhead 2010 Sociology of Religious Emotion. Oxford: Oxford University Press.

Schindler, A. 1999 Angels and the AIDS Epidemic: The Resurgent Popularity of Angel Imagery in the United States of America. Journal of American Culture 22(3):49–61.

Serres, M. 1993 La légende des anges. Paris: Flammarion.

Shilling, C., and P. Mellor 2007 Cultures of Embodied Experience: Technology, Religion and Body Pedagogics. The Sociological Review 55(3):531–549.

Trzebiatowska, M., and S. Bruce 2012 Why Are Women More Religious Than Men? Oxford: Oxford University Press.

Uibu, M. 2013 Creating Meanings and Supportive Networks on the Spiritual Internet Forum 'The Nest of Angels'. Journal of Ethnology and Folkloristics 6:69–86.

Utriainen, T. 2013a Doing Things with Angels: Agency, Alterity and Practices of Enchantment. *In* New Age Spirituality: Rethinking Religion. S. Suttcliffe and I. Gilhus, eds. Pp. 242–255. Durham: Acumen Publishing.

———. 2013b Uskontotaidetta ja enkelinsiipiä: kaksi tapausta suomalaisissa naistenlehdissä. [Art on Religion and Wings of Angels: Two Cases in Finnish Women's Magazines.] Media & Viestintä 2:69–86.

———. 2014 Angels, Agency and Emotions: Global Religion for Women in Finland? *In* Finnish Women Making Religion: Between Ancestors and Angels. T. Utriainen and P. Salmesvuori, eds. Pp. 237–254. New York: Palgrave MacMillan.

———. in press Ritually Framing Enchantment.

Utriainen, T., T. Hovi, and M. Broo 2012 Combining Choice and Destiny: Identity and Agency within Post-Secular Well-being Practices. *In* Post-Secular Society. P. Nynäs, M. Lassander, and T. Utriainen, eds. Pp. 187–216. New Brunswick: Transaction Publishers.

Utriainen, T., and P. Salmesvuori 2014 Finnish Women Making Religion: Between Ancestors and Angels. New York: Palgrave MacMillan.

Verrips, J. 2003 Dr. Jekyll and Mr. Hyde: Modern Medicine Between Magic and Science. *In* Magic and Modernity: Interfaces of Revelation and Concealment. B. Meyer and P. Pels, eds. Pp. 223–240. Stanford: Stanford University Press.

Walter, T. 2011 Angels Not Souls: Popular Religion in the Online Mourning for British Celebrity Jane Goody. Religion 4:29–51.

———. in press The Angelic Dead: Bereavement and Vernacular Religion. Omega: Journal of Death and Dying 73(1).

Wood, M. 2000 Holistic Health Therapies in Comparative Analysis. *In* Healing and Religion. M. Bowman, ed. Pp. 81–94. Middlesex: Hisarlik Press.

Woodhead, L., and E. Sointu 2008 Spirituality, Gender, and Expressive Selfhood. Journal for the Scientific Study of Religion 47:259–276.

# Index

Ackerknecht, E. H., xv, 40, 51–52
Ådahl, S., 243
Adewunmi, A. 201
Adler, S. R., 13
Ae-Ngibise, K., 182
Agha, A., 234
Ahearn, L., 268
Ahlbäck, T., 19
Aina, O. F., 172
Akyeampong, E., 175
Anas, A. A., 183
Andersen, H. M., 172
Andrews, I., 213
Appiah-Kubi, K., 167
Aretaeus, 41
Asad, T., 7
Asuni, T., 201
Aupers, S., 245
Avirappattu, G., 210
Ayim-Aboagye, D., 167
Ayonrinde, O., 201
Baber, Z., 145
Bainbridge, W. S., 120
Banerjee, G., 154
Barbour, I., 12
Barker, I. V., 207
Barker, J., 254
Barnett, H. G., 46
Barrett, D., 207
Barrett, R. J., 49
Bartocci, G., 8
Basu, H., 1–24, 147–149
Beals, A. R., 150
Béhague, D., 22, 182
Belcher, J. R., 209, 212, 214, 220
Bellah, R., 84
Bellamy, C., 145, 148–152, 158
Benedict, R., 8, 47
Bennett, G., 259, 263
Bennett, J., 260
Bentall, R. P., 3
Bercovitch, S., 69–71
Berglund, P. A., 113
Berner, U., 144, 155–156
Bhaskar, H., 150
Bhowmick, K. P., 150
Bhugra, D., 4–6, 111, 154
Bigelow, A. B., 160
Binswanger, L., 90
Birdwell, J., 112

*Index*

Bjorck, J. P., 210–211
Blanch, A., 6
Blankenburg, W., 49
Bloch, E., 145–146
Bloch, M., 123, 217
Blom, J. D., 6
Bobgan, D. and M., 211
Boehnlein, J. K., 10
Bolton, B., 220
Boroffka, A., 189, 201
Bourdieu, P., 156–157
Bourguignon, E., 7, 127
Bowman, M., 253, 257, 260
Brison, K. J., 19
Brodwin, P., 172
Broo, M., 227, 232, 253, 256
Bruce, S., 256
Brugger, W., 10
Bruner, E. M., 230–231
Burman, J. J. R., 146
Calhoun-Brown, A., 7
Campbell, K. K., 268
Campbell-Hall, V., 182
Campion, J., 154
Cannon, D. S., 155
Caroso, C., 92
Carothers, J. C., 5, 39, 61, 190
Casanova, J., 10
Casey, R. L., 220

Castelein, J. D., 220
Celsus, 41
Chappel, P., 210
Chigona, G., 198
Chilivumbo, A. B., 193
Chiu, M., 210
Clarke, B., 42–43
Clifford, J., 23
Cohen, A., 4
Cohn, N., xvi
Cole, E. 112
Comaroff, J. and J. L., 196
Conrad, P., 22
Cook, C. C. H., 13
Cooper, J. E., 41, 45–46
Corin, E., 15, 89–109, 199, 201
Corten, A., 19
Cotton, J., 76
Cox, H., 207, 211–212
Crapanzano, V., 89, 104
Csordas, T. J., 2, 6, 8, 10, 17, 127–139, 211, 216–217, 260, 266–267
Czihak, G., 60
Dahla, B., 19
Dana, R. H., 220
Darwin, C., 57
David, A. M., 146
Davies, D., 112, 123

Dayton, D. W., 211
De Gordon, B., 42
De Jong, J. T. V. M., 6, 8
Dein, S., 2, 4, 19, 50, 159, 207–219
Deleuze, G., 231
Dennis-Antwi, J. A., 183
Desjarlais, R. R., 245
Devereux, G., xv, 9, 40–41, 47–48, 51–52
Diethelm, O., 41–42
Dobbins, R., 207–208
Domino, G., 113
Doniger, W., 107
Draper, S., 254–255
Dumont, L., 80–81, 107
Durkheim, É., 15, 67, 78, 85, 118, 123, 241
Dwyer, G., 150
Edgerton, R., 8
Edwards, L., 211
Ehrenberg, A., 15, 18, 67–85, 268
Eliade, M., 39
Ellis, S., 191
Emerson, R. W., 70–71
Engelke, M., 218
Englund, H., 199
Erichsen, C., 61
Eriksen, A., 218
Erikson, E. H., 47–48, 62, 73
Ernst, C., 153
Ernst, W., 4
Evans, R., 41–42
Evans-Pritchard, E. E., 37, 62, 81
Fabrega, H., 49
Favret-Saada, J., 9
Fedida, P., 109
Feierman, S., 167–168, 172
Feyerabend, P. K., 62
Fiedler, K., 199
Field, M., 40, 45, 167
Firth, R., 46
Flueckiger, J. B., 149–150, 159
Flum, M. E., 210
Fortes, M., 40
Fortune, R., 8
Fosu, G. B., 167
Foucault, M., 4, 22, 67
Francis, L. J., 120
Frank, J. and J., 127–128
Frazer, J. G., 39
Freud, S., 3, 8, 38, 61, 72–73, 82, 119, 234, 246
Fulford, K. W. M., 6, 11
Gadamer, H-G., 157
Gaines, A. D., 22
Galen, 41–42

*Index*

Gardella, P., 254–255
Garrison, V., 89, 104
Gauthier, A., 91–92
Geertz, C., 48
Geschiere, P., 179
Gilbert, M., 175
Gilhus, I. S., 254–255
Gilman, S., 5, 190
Gilmartin, D., 145, 152
Glock, C. Y., 155
Goddard, M., 8
Good, B. J., 10–12
Goodwin, G., 71
Gorsuch, R., 210
Gottschalk, P., 145, 152–153, 155
Graveling, E., 170
Griffith, R., 210–211
Gritzmacher, S. A., 220
Gunther Brown, C., 200, 207, 212, 215–216
Gupta, S., 6
Gureje, O., 181, 201
Habermas, J., 10
Haeckel, E., 60
Hager, M., 128
Hall, S. M., 209, 212, 214, 220
Halliburton, M., 142, 182
Halliday, A., 39

Hamilton, M., 215
Hammond, F. and I. M., 210
Hampshire, K. R., 182–183
Hanks, W. F., 229, 231
Hawthorne, H., 46
Heclo, H., 10
Heelas, P., 7, 13, 210, 237, 245
Hegde, R., 145–146
Heinz, A., 14, 57–64, 201
Herle, A., 37
Hervieu-Léger, D., 13
Hippocrates, 41–42
Hodgson, M., 152
Holloman, R., 237
Honko, L., 233
Hopper, K., 39–41
Horton, R., 171
Horwitz, A., 22
Hoskins, 46
Houtman, D., 245
Hovi, T., 227, 232, 253, 256
Howells, W. W., 7
Huber, S., 155
Huguelet, P., 6
Hunt, S., 215
Hunter, R., 39, 42–43
Ibbetson, J., 144
Incayawar, R., 12
Ingstad, B., 183

Jablensky, A., 41
Jadhav, S., 6, 178
Jain, S., 178
Jenkins, J. H., 4–6, 23, 135
Jeste, D. V., 41
Jilek, W. G., 3
Johannsen, H., 128
Johnson, T., 207
Jones, J. W., 6
Jorm, A., 210
Josephson, A. M., 10
Jung, C. G., 38–39
Kaiser, P., 6
Kakar, S., 151
Kalu, O., 200
Karayanni, M. M., 10
Kaspin, D., 196
Keane, W., 231
Kendall, L., 10
Keppens, M., 145–146
Kessler, R., 113
Kiev, A., 127
Kilns, R., 41–42
King, M., 114, 122, 145
Kircher, T. T. J., 50–51
Kirmayer, L. J., 5–6, 9, 14, 189, 199, 201
Kis-Halas, J., 254–255
Kitanaka, J., 67
Kivivuori, J., 231
Kleinman, A., 5–6, 11, 127–128
Koenig, H. G., 6, 220
Konadu, K., 167
Konkka, U., 230, 234, 241
Koski, K., 234, 243
Kraepelin, E., 3–4, 8, 39
Krause, K., 218
Kray, C. A., 19
Kuhn, T. S., 62
La Barre, W., 45, 47–48, 52
La Fontaine, J. S., 196, 198
Laderman, C., 6
Lafuze, J., 210
Lambek, M., 104, 107
Lambo, T. A., 39, 201
Lasch, C., 69, 71, 75, 77
Lassander, M., 253
Last, M., 168
Latour, B., 12, 20, 23, 253
Lau, R. W. K., 229, 238
Laubscher, B., 44
Laurinkiené, N., 243
Lauzon, G., 91
Lawal, R., 201
Lawrence, B. B., 145, 152
Lazar, I., 128
Leavey, G., 2, 16, 19, 111–124
Leckie, J., 22

*Index*

Leff, J., 40
Lehmann, D., 8, 10
Leighton, A. H., 201
Leube, D. T., 50–51
LeVine, R. A., 197
Lévi-Strauss, C., 3, 62
Lewis, D., 216
Lewis, S., 177
Lewton, E., 127
Lieberman, J., 177
Lienhardt, G., 37, 51
Lim, R., 11
Lindfors, P., 264
Lindhardt, M., 217
Lindholm, C., 229
Lipsedge, M., 6
Littler, M., 112
Littlewood, R., xv–xvii, 4–6, 8, 14–15, 37–52
Lock, A., 210
Lock, M., 22
Locke, J., 42, 215
Loewenthal, K., 122
Lorenzen, D. N., 145
Louden, S. H., 120
Luckmann, T., 260, 266
Luedke, T. J., 8, 218
Luhrmann, T. M., 9, 22, 216, 219, 260, 262–263, 266, 269

Lwanda, J. L. C., 193
Macalpine, I., 39, 42–43
MacDonald, M., 41–42
MacLachlan, M., 193
MacNutt, F., 210, 213
Madan, T. N., 107
Mahone, S., 5, 190
Makari, G., 73
Malinowski, B., 3, 37–38
Mandelbaum, D., 147, 150, 153
Marriott, M., 19
Marshall-Fratani, R., 19
Marwick, M. G., 193
Mascia-Lees, F., 138
Mason, K., 122
Mauss, M., 9, 68, 72, 82
Maxwell, D., 19
Mayer, D. Y., 40
Mayers, C., 113
McBride, P., 114
McCabe, R., 112
McCall, J. C., 172
McCaskie, T. C., 169, 171
McClay, W. M., 10
McClure, R., 210
McCulloch, J., 5, 61, 190
McDaniel, J., 7
McDougall, W., 38
McGrath, J., 41–42

McGuire, M., 253
McKindley-Alverez, C., 210
McPherson, J., 253, 264
Meador, K., 220
Meyer, B., 9, 19, 168, 218, 253
Minas, H., 5
Minkus, H. K., 174
Mönter, N., 57
Moodley, R., 128
Morel, B. A., 58
Morris, B., 183, 197–198, 201
Mueller, T., 4
Mullings, L., 167
Murken, S., 254, 266
Murphy, H. B. M., 40, 48
Murphy, J., 48
Nadel, S. F., 39
Nandy, A., 151
Napier, R., 42
Naraindas, H., 5, 13, 147
Needham, R., 11
Nichter, M., 6
Nunley, M., 6
Nyando, C., 193–194
Nyirenda, T., 193–194
Nynäs, P., 253
Obeng, P., 175
Oberoi, H., 144
Offiong, D. A., 182

Ohlmarks, C. A., 46
Olusoga, D., 61
Orr, D. M. R., 182
Orsi, R., 253, 259
Owusu, S. A., 182–183
Padel, R., 41
Padmavati, R., 15, 89–109
Pandey, G., 146
Pankow, A., 14, 57–64
Parry, J., 123
Patel, V., 177, 182
Pattison, E. M., 220
Peglidou, A., 170
Pels, P., 9, 253
Peltzer, K., 189, 193–194
Perkins, D., 210
Peteet, J. R., 10
Pfeiffer, M., 3
Philo, 41
Pickett, K., 68
Pigg, S. L., 172
Pinard, S., 216
Pohjanheimo, O., 253
Poloma, M. M., 209, 213, 220
Porcello, T., 216
Porter, R., 2, 5
Porterfield, A., 211
Powell, R., 39
Priebe, S., 112

*Index*

Prince, M., 8
Prince, R., 201
Probst, P., 196
Prochaska, F., 120
Putnam, R. D., 74
Quack, 5, 17, 141–161
Racamier, P., 105, 107
Read, U. M., 2, 17–18, 167–184
Reddy, W. M., 235
Reich, W., 62
Rieff, P., 75–76
Riesman, D., 72
Riis, O., 258
Rivers, W. H., 38
Robbins, J., 19, 217
Roberts, C., 210
Roberts, S. R., 233
Romanucci-Ross, L., 170
Rondon, J., 114
Rose, N., 8–9, 13, 227–228, 231
Roseman, M., 6
Rosen, G., 41
Rouse, S., 37
Roy, S., 154
Ruthven, J., 209
Sadler, Z., 11
Sadowsky, J., 4, 201
Salmesvuori, P., 256
Sartorius, N., 41, 45–46

Sass, L., 49–52
Sax, W., 5, 8, 20, 146–147, 150
Schindler, A., 268–269
Schmalz, M., 145
Schmidt, L. E., 215
Schoffeleers, M., 192
Schumaker, J. F., 1, 6
Scull, A., 22
Sébastia, B., 147, 153
Seligman, C. G., 4, 37–39, 44, 52
Sennett, R., 69, 71, 75–77
Seremetakis, N., 216
Serres, M., 255
Shils, E., 74–75
Shirokogoroff, S. M., 63
Shorter, E., 2, 10
Silverman, J., 6, 39
Simon, B., 41
Skultans, V., 6, 158
Smart, N., 155
Smith, B., 231, 239
Smith, D. J., 218
Sointu, E., 265
Soranus, 41
Springer, K., 213
Stack, S., 118
Stark, R., 120, 155
Steinforth, A. S., 1–24, 189–202

Stepanova, E., 233–234
Stewart, T., 153
Stocking, G., 37–38
Stoller, P., 216
Strathern, M., 19, 167
Stroeken, K., 168, 183
Strohbehn, U., 199
Stubbe, H., 190
Styers, R., 9
Sue, D. W. and D., 210
Taetzsch, W. J., 210
Taylor, C., 9, 122–123, 230
Tempels, P., 198
Ter Haar, G., 191
Thiessen, H., 208
Thomas, J. C., 214
Thornicroft, G., 177, 182
Tocqueville, A. de, 71, 79–80, 84
Tolbert, E., 234–235, 241, 248–249
Torrey, E. F., 39
Trice, P. D., 210–211
Trilling, L., 228, 230, 235, 240
Trzebiatowska, M., 256
Turner, R. H., 75
Turner, V. W., 104, 167, 183
Tutkimuskeskus, K., 254
Uibu, M., 254, 258

Uomoto, J., 210
Urban, G., 248
Utriainen, T., 2, 20, 227, 232, 253–269
Van der Veer, P., 151, 153, 160
Van Dijk, R., 199
Van Ommeren, M., 6, 8
Vaughan, M., 5
Ventevogel, P., 183
Verhagen, P. J., 10–13
Verrips, J., 253
Village, A., 211
Wachtel, P. L., 245
Wacker, G., 210, 215
Wakefield, J., 22
Wald, K. D., 7
Waldram, J., 128
Wallace, E. R., 38
Walter, T., 215, 254, 258
Wang, P. S., 113
Wang, N., 230–231
Warrington, K., 213
Weaver, A. J., 113, 120
Weber, M., 9, 71
Weinhold, J., 8
Weis, H. M., 112
West, H. G., 8, 218
West, W., 128
Wheelis, A., 73

*Index*

Whitehouse, H., 155
Whitley, R., 6
Whyte, S. R., 22, 168, 171
Wiesenfeld, A. R., 112
Wilce, J. M., 2, 19, 22, 227–249
Wilkinson, R. G., 68
Williams, F. E., 45
Williams, J., 213
Willis, T., 43
Wilson, B., 47
Wimber, J., 213, 215
Winch, P., 81
Wing, J., 41, 45–46
Wintrob, R., 13
Wishlade, R. L., 196
Wittgenstein, L., 78–79
Wood, M., 253, 257, 259, 265, 269
Woodhead, L., 258, 265
Yang, L. H., 183
Young, A., 3, 22, 159
Young, D., 39
Zilboorg, G., 41
Zimmerman, F., 67